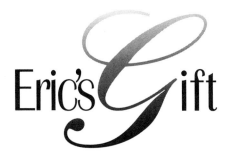

Eric's Gift

by
Kimberly Thompson

*A mother's discovery of unconditional love
in the 47th chromosome*

For all the doctors and nurses who saved my baby's life, who loved him and mended him while he healed and grew.

Some of the names in this book have been changed in honor of maintaining privacy.

For requests to have
the author speak to your organization
or to share your reflections, please
email or send a note to the addresses below.

Published by
Eric's Gift Enterprises
P.O. Box 340516
Tampa, Florida 33694

ericsgift@aol.com

http://www.ericsgift.com

Library of Congress Catalog Card No.: 98-93202
ISBN: 0-9665250-3-5

Printed and bound in the United States of America

Acknowledgment

This book is an acknowledgment of the extraordinary people who have supported and loved me and my family during these growing and healing times.

I must first acknowledge my son, Eric, who has given me more life than I gave to him.

To my husband, Bob, whose true love and partnership and determination to live his dreams keeps me inspired and loving him every day.

To Stacy, who listened from her heart every time I read another chapter and who hugged me on the beach when I couldn't bear reading the chapter I had just written; who listened, read, edited, talked me through the rough chapters, and giggled with me through the funny ones.

To Jonathan, without whose conversations none of this would have been possible.

To Mark and Genie, who showed up in my life just when I needed them. They came whenever I asked, they supported us without question, they learned with us about how to take care of Eric, they were always close by and, though they have moved far away, remain close — in my heart.

To Patti, a long-time friend, who walked miles with me, talking and listening and always finding the rainbow in the rain.

To Tom and Sharon for refreshing our lives with their visits.

To Mom and Dad, whose love for me and my baby moves me to tears.

Foreword

The Beginnings of *Eric's Gift*

I remember the day she told us she was going to write her story. It seemed so right; a moment when another piece of life's puzzle fell into place and fit—perfectly. And she asked me to work with her, to help her edit and so forth (as if you could edit a heart, I thought, but didn't say so). It was as though she were handing me her child and asking me to decide what features it would have—tall, short, blue eyes or brown, friendly, shy...so many details, choices, decisions. It seemed too much for my hands. So rather than holding her child, I held her heart and asked it to keep uncovering itself so others could see. To keep giving of itself, unchanged. Yes, eventually the words of the heart got edited a bit, but the heart never did. And here in this book, her heart is given intimately, hilariously, unselfishly to ours.

BY STACY CLARK

Preface

Eric's Gift began as *A Mother's Journey* in October of 1993. My son, Eric, was on life support, battling pneumonia with collapsed lungs and a damaged heart, and the doctors questioned whether he would live. I wanted to remember what it felt like to be a mother; the sense of not being able to distinguish where my flesh ended and his began when I pressed my cheek against his, when the warmth of our energies connected and calmed my fears. I wanted to remember the wisp of curls that twirled behind his ears and the feeling of "life fulfilled" when his eyes drifted to look into mine. Mostly, I wanted to remember that unexplainable warmth in my heart when I held him, thought of him, talked about him or just touched him. How could I remember the feeling of being of mother, when it looked as though it would only last two months?

I decided I would write it down—write everything, so I wouldn't, couldn't forget.

From that moment, words, sentences, paragraphs flooded my thoughts. Effortlessly, I began formulating and structuring chapters in my mind interlaced between conversations, before slipping off to sleep, upon waking, while driving and at Eric's bedside. During Eric's second week on life support, I strode up the cement walkway leading to the hospital entrance, past the reception desk to the bank of elevators, all the while forming our evening strolls together into sentences. As I stood in the bare hallway in silent anticipation, waiting to see my son, I gazed upward to the yellow numbers blinking too slowly on 5, then 4, 3, then 2 and finally 1. As the grand steel doors parted for me, I smiled at the grandparents, nurses and orderly and stepped into the elevator as though it were the entrance to an evening ball. Leaning against the icy cold wall, I quickly relaxed back into my sanctuary of words as the elevator crept upward seven floors to the children's ward.

Before my husband got to the hospital that night, I told Eric about writing the book, quietly, sheepishly, so no one else would hear. It was to be our secret and the book would be for him and me only. By the time Bob arrived, I remembered that I don't keep secrets, especially at a time when opening up and expressing concerns seemed essential. I decided I would just tell Bob and our very close friends, Jonathan and Stacy.

When I made my announcement to the three of them, it took me saying the words twice—louder the second time—for them to hear me fully and completely, but when they did, a sweet silence blanketed the room. Looking back, I believe it was a blanket woven with love. With open hearts, they agreed to be my support (there was no question, but I had to ask); Stacy with her editing skills, Jonathan with his coaching abilities and Bob with his love.

A Mother's Journey became a compulsion. I began writing that evening at my kitchen table occasionally catching a glimpse of the empty cradle in the living room. The journey, thank God, carried us through the life support crisis and over the next two years as Eric dangled his legs over death's pier, the water splashing up onto his toes and tickling his backside. With each emergency and breakthrough, I wrote our experience, transformation and insights, peeling away fears and inner obstacles that very gradually opened up life so it became lighter, richer and fulfilling to a level that I never knew was possible. Somewhere in the middle of the two years, I found myself sitting at the large table in the corner room of the Unity Center where we held our *Up With Downs* meetings. I was across from a new mom and dad, brand new. She held her month-old, blond-haired Down syndrome infant against her chest, protectively and lovingly, while her husband wrung his hands in his lap. "We haven't told our parents yet," she said. My eyes were transfixed on the young father's face while she spoke. His tears never stopped. It came to me as I watched him, *Eric's Gift* would not be a secret. The book would not be for just Eric and me or just our close friends and family. *Eric's Gift* would be for anyone and everyone. *Eric's Gift* would help this man embrace his infant son and his life and cherish unexpected challenges.

The day I knew *A Mother's Journey* was complete was when the journey unveiled the essence of the book and the title transformed into *Eric's Gift*. It was a gift from my son, a gift I now know was always there. His smile, his warmth, his being gently revealed the gift so that I could see it for myself and share with others. *Eric's Gift* comes to you from my heart and from Eric's repaired heart that after four and one half years continues to beat louder and stronger with every passing moment. With love and miracles, our hearts beat with yours.

Spring 1998
KAT

Every person,
all the events of your life
are there because you have
drawn them there.

What you choose
to do with them is
up to you.

Richard Bach
ILLUSIONS

His 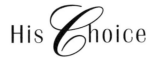hoice

October 1993

The phone rang, 11 p.m. as planned.

"Hi, Mark," my husband, uttered, knowing it was Mark on the line.

"Hi, Bob," Mark replied softly, while Genie's cheerier, yet somewhat heavy-hearted "Hi!" spoke out from a second telephone. They were friends who had grown into becoming our earthbound guardian angels since our baby was born: watching us, helping us, listening to us, calling us at any moment we needed them, even when we weren't sure if we did, and when we were just plain at a loss. Married just a few months when we met them during my second trimester, they were a team who instantly gave us their friendship and their love.

"I'm here, too," I said anxiously anticipating the conversation that was about to begin.

"Lew is holding. Let me conference him in," Mark said, referring to his uncle in California.

The phone clicked a couple times, and then Lew Epstein's resounding voice bellowed into my ear, "Hello, my children." His greeting struck me as odd—I had never been referred to as "my children" before. Nevertheless, I listened on.

1

I had never met this man, but Mark and Genie had told us of his life's work. During his 75 years, he has produced many tapes and workshops on such topics as the gift of babies, intimacy in relationships and "listening that you are loved." I knew his commitment to love and his ability to fully express love would somehow give me solace while, Eric, my two-month-old baby, lay in an intensive care unit (ICU) crib, being fed through tubes and kept alive by a life support machine. I knew this man had connections to hundreds of people worldwide, and my intention on this phone call was to ask him to have everyone he could reach align, intend and pray together to have Eric gain in health—more truthfully, to live.

I recognized Lew's voice from the tapes and heard the familiar tone of love. He was talking to two people who hadn't seen their baby open his eyes for two weeks, a baby who lay still and limp through constant sedation and paralyzing drugs.

We were not allowed to hold Eric or rock him, only to caress his frail arms and to gently hold his lifeless hands. Even a kiss on the cheek could disturb the breathing tube. I comforted him with my voice, telling him tales of what our life would be like together. I told him about the zoo and all its playful animals. I told him about picnics we would have and what it's like to swing high. I promised to "push" until he had had enough. I told him about building sand castles and rolling in the break of waves. I sang *You Are My Sunshine* and *House at Pooh Corner* through tears that I could not suppress. I spent hours holding his little fingers, reading my favorite books to him, wondering if his young spirit could soar as high as *Jonathan Livingston Seagull*, if my baby's will to live equaled the strength and determination of the young seagull. I shared Winnie the Pooh's wisdom in *The Tao of Pooh* and explained who Pooh and Piglet and Christopher Robin were. I pleaded with him to stay.

What I hadn't done is what Lew Epstein now asked me: "Have you told Eric where he is? Have you explained to him his medical problems and told him what Down syndrome is?"

"No," I replied, taken aback. It had never occurred to me to tell Eric his situation. What could he do? Why would I tell him?

"He needs to know his situation so he can make a choice," Lew said. A choice?

What choice? No, no! And then my heart sank upon hearing that it could be up to Eric whether to stay or not, whether to live or to die. I didn't want to give him that choice. I had already chosen for both of us, all of us, that he would live, live a long, full, happy life. I couldn't give that up. I couldn't let him choose. What if he chose to go? No, I won't let him go. My stomach knotted and my hands shook with resistance as I gripped the receiver ever tighter.

Lew told us of his own experience with his four-month-old child dying of Sudden Infant Death Syndrome. Even at 75, his memory of that special baby was clear, and the teaching that baby provided in his short life, so many years ago, continues. Lew told us he was sorry for what we were going through, his manifest love for humanity pouring out with every word.

I broke down into the phone as he spoke; he was so absolute. But with each tear, I began to gradually, slowly let go of the control over my baby's life. The more Lew spoke, the more I let go. In my heart, his words rang true for me. I realized that it was truly Eric's choice to live or die, and that he could choose either. My heart broke open with the thought of losing him now. It is too soon. He's too young.

3

He hasn't had the chance to enjoy life yet and I haven't had a chance to be a mother. My heart ached to hold him and comfort him and somehow make him stay with me.

"It's Eric's life, and he has to make the choice," Lew said, weeping, his words piercing my heart. "I'm so sorry, my child." My illusion of control over Eric's life slipped away with every passing thought. I was sad, yet somehow relieved. As he continued to speak, I was becoming free of a burden that I now knew I couldn't have carried anyway. Although my mind resisted, my heart was letting go. I could give him the choice; it was rightfully his to make anyway. And along with handing over something that never belonged to me in the first place, I would let him know how much I loved him and how much I respected his decision, but how, with every part of my body and soul, I wanted him to live.

After nearly an hour passed, my eyes were dry and the conversation came to a close. Even though a thank you seemed almost trite given what had just transpired, we thanked Lew, Mark and Genie and said our goodbyes.

I was certain about what I needed to do, as was Bob. It was after midnight. Nurse's change of shift reporting would be over by now, which meant parents were allowed back into ICU.

We drove to the hospital in silence, reliving the conversation we'd just had. Over and over again I heard Lew say, "tell him everything, he needs to know everything to make a choice."

After calling into ICU for permission to enter, then stopping at the washbasin to sterilize our hands, we positioned ourselves on either side of Eric's crib, each gently taking a hand into ours. We told him of his current plight, describing the machines, the tubes, the treatments, the medicines, his heart condition, all about Down syndrome, and our feelings. We shared with him our sadness, and just how scary this all was for us. We told him everything. I wanted to make sure he had all the facts and all the feelings so he'd be well-informed for his decision.

Hours passed. We were drained and exhausted. There was nothing left to tell, at least for now, and it was time to go. I raised Eric's tiny hand and kissed it softly. I walked backward from his bed, watching him, wondering, hoping that this wasn't the last time I would see my baby alive.

CHAPTER TWO

Eric's 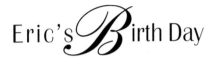irth Day

August 22, 1993

It was a Sunday, thirty-six weeks into my pregnancy. I was larger than I had ever been in my life. I waddled instead of walked, the soles of my feet ached with every step, my fingers throbbed with every bend, and this morning brought something new: I was uncontrollably peeing in spurts every ten minutes.

"What's this?" my mind asked.

Unfortunately the answer came from the same mind, "I have no idea."

"Okay, I'll nonchalantly mention it to Bob and see if he acts concerned," I said to myself, "if not, we'll go to breakfast with Patti and Ernie as planned."

"Sounds good," I replied silently.

Off to the toilet I went for the fourth or fifth time this morning.

"Hey Bob, something weird is happening," I exclaimed to a sleeping husband. The news barely stirred him. After eight months he was used to my daily reports of the changes in my body. "I keep peeing and I can't stop it."

"Hmmm," he moaned, "Does it look strange?"

"No, looks normal to me."

"Well, if it keeps happening we can call the doctor when

we get back from breakfast."

"Okay." Once again my nerves were calmed.

"The Brunchery" was just across the street. I didn't notice any more unwanted spurts during the brief walk. "Everything is fine," my mind whispered reassuringly.

It was 10:30 a.m. and today was our last chance to spend time with our friend Ernie. He had to be on his way back to Atlanta on a 1 p.m. flight.

I met Ernie and Patti twelve years ago when we were all budding, new airmen right out of the United States Air Force basic training. Over the years, Ernie and I had lost touch, but Patti's letters kept us both up to date on each others' lives. As fate would have it, after the years in the Air Force, Patti moved to Tampa, followed by Ernie a couple of years later, followed by me a couple more years later. Unfortunately, just two weeks after my move, Ernie was transferred to Atlanta.

"Hey guys!" Ernie yelled from the back of the restaurant. He and Patti were already seated at a table and waiting for us.

Seeing Patti's waving hand, I recalled watching that hand fluff her curly, auburn mane as she was getting ready to go out on a date. I was a mere eighteen, shy and naive, while she at twenty-three, was a woman of the world. I listened in awe to her stories about her treks in Greece, her college exploits in San Francisco, and the exotic men that she had dated. She was full of life, a A go-getter, prepared to tackle anything that came her way.

After we settled in, we chatted over the menus for a while and ordered. There were only three trips to the bathroom during that 15-minute block. I could tell everyone was wondering what was going on with me, but I didn't say anything and neither did they. They must have figured they were pregnancy-related incidents.

It finally struck me. There I was locked in the men's room (The women's room was occupied and, as pregnant women will understand, I couldn't wait!), my mind racing through every emotion: fear, excitement, joy, uncertainty, embarrassment, nervousness, silliness and even a little melancholy that the pregnancy was coming to an end. I giggled to myself and stopped short with an "Oh my God!"

Back to the table I went with the sheepish grin one gets when she has a secret and is reveling in the thought of telling someone. I sat down quietly, knowingly. Our meals had been served and my companions were voraciously digging into their omelets. I couldn't contain my excitement. I grinned widely and let out an abrupt snicker. They all looked up at me still awkwardly shoveling in the bacon and muffins.

"My water broke!" I blurted out.

The three of them stopped all movement. I was reminded of the *Twilight Zone* episode where all the people became mannequins except, of course, the one poor soul who was chosen to go crazy during that half hour.

Dad-to-be was tongue-tied, although I saw the sides of his mouth begin to curl up. Ernie was dumbfounded and soon-to-be Aunt Patti broke the silence.

"What does this mean?" she asked wide-eyed with a shaky voice.

"It means we're going to have a baby today!" I said now giggling openly, more comfortable with the idea.

Still frozen, their eyes darted to each other and back to me. Once again, Patti's was the only voice to speak. She asked cautiously, "Should we go to the hospital now?"

Funny she should ask me, as if I was supposed to know. None of us at the table had ever had a baby before, so why ask me? I thought back to all the "labor and delivery" conversations I'd had with Mom, Janine, my older sister, and all of my mom-friends and wondered, "why didn't I know my water broke and why don't I know what to do." Did they never tell me or is it simply impossible for a non-mother to have heard what they were saying? I can only recall smiling blankly and nodding pointlessly as they droned on and on about their experiences. My thoughts would drift to "Why are they telling me all of this? Is it time to leave? Where should I go shopping? Geez, I wish my hair would grow out...." I would be lost to them for the rest of the conversation.

But now it was time for a decision and I could tell I was appointed decision-maker by default. I did recall the instructor, in my second and last prenatal class, saying it was okay to relax at home for a while after water breakage since we could be trapped in a hospital room in labor for hours. Taking her advice, and more importantly, satisfying my hunger, I suggested we finish breakfast and then go to the hospital. From that moment on the plan unfolded. The mannequins came to life, breathing deeply and somewhat relieved by my lack of urgency. Consuming continued. I dug into my bland eggs Benedict with crabmeat, considering the hours that may lapse before I got to eat again. As a team we developed a sure-fire plan to be carried out after breakfast.

1. Patti goes home to get her portable stereo so that I can listen to soothing Native American flute music during labor (Right!).
2. Ernie taxis to the airport, calls Patti at home for the telephone number of St. Joseph's Women's Hospital and calls again for a status check when he lands in Atlanta.
3. Bob and I walk home and put together an overnight bag

4. I call Dr. Mazor to ensure the time is near (four more visits to the restroom still didn't completely convince us).
5. Bob and I drive to the hospital and Patti meets us there by 1 p.m.

Once home, Bob snapped into action. He found the pre-written checklist in the mess of papers from the prenatal class and began his search. I sat on the bed watching him with amusement. First the overnight bag, but which one? The ugly green one with the brown strap? No, it's torn inside. Okay, how about the blue one with the long gray strap? Nope, has his workout clothes in it already. He settled on the gray and pink nylon bag. Good choice. Next, he grabbed my bathrobe, my slippers, and began rummaging through my drawers for more items on the checklist.

"What else, what else," he said to himself a little exasperated and a lot excited.

Meanwhile, I put a call into Dr. Mazor's answering service.

While I waited for the doctor to call back, I phoned my sister to confirm water breakage. After two natural births I thought she'd recognize the signs.

"Yep," she said, "it sounds like he's ready to come out."

"But, he's not due for another month. We're not ready."

She laughed comfortingly. "Doesn't matter, *he's* ready." She teased me a little about what I was about to go through and told me she loved me. *Big sisters are wonderful!*

The doctor called back within five minutes.

"Meet me at the hospital immediately," he directed gently.

"But the instructor said I could stay at home until the contractions came every ten minutes." My naiveté was showing.

"I don't know why they would tell you that, it's not right," he continued, "at least one baby has died at birth from waiting at home. Don't wait. Come in right away and I'll meet you there."

"Okay, we'll be there in ten minutes." He heard no arguments from me. Bob was still walking briskly back and forth, stopping in mid-stride to turn and look at me with wondering, loving eyes and a smile full of pride and love. Back to work. He darted from room to room, closet to dresser, and back again never letting go of that precious checklist. We knew this was it and he was carrying out his "husbandly duties" quite thoroughly, each item checked off on the list as collected. He flipped the paper over and looked up at me perplexed.

"The baby," he said duped. "We forgot about stuff for the baby."

Since the baby chose to enter this world a month early, we were very ill-prepared. Not only hadn't we prepared an overnight bag for me, we barely had anything to even collect for the baby. The nursery was still a photography room newly decorated with a jungle animal lamp, an empty changing table, a baby "snoozer" swing, and lastly, the quintessential car seat.

"I'll grab some diapers, a couple blankets, the car seat and let's go," Bob said hurriedly.

"One more quick call to make before we go," I requested. "I've got to call Dad."

"Okay, hurry," he demanded sweetly.

Dad had adamantly urged me to call him the minute I went into labor. He wanted to be with me when the baby was born. He had two hours to drive and was more ready to go than we were.

"Hello" he said, accent on the first syllable like it was

any other normal day.

"Hi Grandpa!" I exclaimed. He knew who it was immediately and sensed my excitement. "Guess what?"

"You're in labor?" he guessed. I could feel his joy and see his smile across the phone line. "I'm leaving now," and he hung up. No time for goodbyes. Next time I see him I'll be a mother. What a funny thought—he always held the title of parent, now it's my turn. Something else to bind us.

He had missed both of my sister's deliveries almost ten years ago and was committed to being a part of mine, which I was thrilled about. Mom had also missed Janine's pregnancies.

After he and my mom were divorced in 1979, the family went in their own directions: Mom to Michigan, Dad stayed in Florida, Janine to Ohio, and me to Texas with the Air Force. Mom has since moved back to Florida with her second husband of thirteen years, just thirty minutes away from Dad and two hours from me. Since we moved to Florida a year ago, Mom and Dad have rekindled an old friendship for my sake and the sake of our new baby. Now they can be with us together without awkwardness, animosity or hurtful hearts. It's wonderful how new lives can heal old wounds. They've been beside themselves watching *their* skinny daughter grow bigger and bigger in anticipation of a new life in our family. Yes, our family. We are a family. We have formed and reformed bonds that not even a divorce can destroy. Grandpa plans to take the baby to the beach, give him his first ride on the motorcycle (a little later), while Grandma shops for him, cuddles him, and teaches him to say Mama. Between Bob's and my estranged families, the baby will have five grandpas, two great-grandpas, four grandmas, and one great-grandma. Love was certainly one thing our baby would get plenty of. BABY.....WOW!

I stood up from the bed and I was suddenly knocked back down. My belly, once flat and acceptable for a two-piece bikini, squeezed and tightened until it was hard as a basketball.

"Oh, my God, I think I'm having a contraction...Bob!...Help!" I yelled so loudly that not only did Bob hear it on the first take, but the neighbors in the next apartment probably did also.

"BREATHE!" came from the baby's room as footsteps pounded their way to my side.

I did as instructed and I remembered the meditations we did during sunsets on St. Pete Beach. Deep breath, in through the nose and out through the mouth. And again. The tightness subsided, my basketball transformed into a beach ball as I continued to relax.

My bags were packed, the house was semi-clean, the baby's room was in complete disarray and we were off.

He stopped me before stepping over the threshold. His hands were around my waist. His eyes pierced deeply into mine.

"I love you," he whispered, tears welling in his eyes, a tender smile dancing on his lips.

"I love you," I whispered back matching his tears and smile. We kissed softly, lovingly, knowing we were stepping into a new adventure together. Together. The clock stopped ticking and we united, sharing the past eight years, the present moment, and our uncertain future simultaneously. Acknowledged through a look and a kiss, we are soulmates, now not only linked by love, but also linked by life. A new life, one we created. One that would never have been if we hadn't found each other in that tiny village in Germany almost ten years ago.

My world had changed in that hallway next to the water

fountain — the moment I first laid eyes on him and couldn't unlay them. He was the most handsome man I had ever seen. He was friendly and confident, and charmed me instantly with his humor. His opening line, "between me, you and the fencepost" wouldn't make it at the *Improv*, but I was captivated. He shared with me a secret about his upcoming trip to Bavaria and we didn't even know each other. I smiled and listened.

We ended up going on that trip to Bavaria together and have been together ever since. For two years we played together in our playground abroad: skiing in the German Alps, sipping mint tea in Tangiers, sharing pitchers of sangria in Lloret de Mar, Spain, and finally marrying in Basel, Switzerland.

I called him my male counterpart since the very beginning. I knew in my heart we would share an incredible life together.

It was a straight shot to the hospital, ten minutes if we hit all the green lights, twelve minutes give or take a few red ones. The squeeze of another contraction came, this time even stronger. I writhed in the passenger's seat, no where to go for comfort and nothing to do for the pain. My throat constricted; only guttural moans slipped through. "This really hurts," I said surprised! I was shocked by the intensity of the contraction and then I was shocked that I was shocked. How is it that billions and billions of women have given birth and I didn't have a clue as to how much it hurt? A well-kept secret was my only answer. I knew there would be more to come.

He drove faster.

In between contractions, a peaceful silence permeated the car. I suppose he may have been contemplating how life was about to change.

He zipped into the privileged parking lot (deliveries only) of St. Joseph's Women's Hospital. We knew what to expect regarding the rooms. Just two weeks ago we had spent a couple of hours in a labor room—I hadn't felt those comforting baby kicks in more than twelve hours, which frightened me enough to call the doctor. He had sent me to this hospital and had ordered a test to monitor the baby's movements. The spikes on the printout had confirmed his kicks, punches and rolls even when I couldn't feel them. The baby turned out to be fine. Nothing to be concerned about. We had been sent home reassured. Now we were back.

It was a slow delivery day at St. Joe's. There was only one other car in the lot. The scene seemed typical. Husband helps wife out of car because wife is incapable of getting out herself. Holding the overnight bag with one hand, husband assists wife across the lot, through the automatic doors and to the front desk. Guard at front door smiles knowingly — he's seen this scene a thousand times before. Receptionist detains us for just a few minutes with the formalities. Nurse comes to escort us to our room and smack! I was hit with the most painful contraction yet. My arm flew to the counter bracing me. I doubled over and cried aloud. I was at the mercy of my body. I was a shoe-in for an epidural. Bob held me tightly, softly saying comforting phrases; we both knew there was nothing he could do.

"Keep breathing," he whispered. "It's okay. We're almost to the room and then you can lie down. Are you okay? Will you make it? Keep breathing. Hold onto me. Are you okay?"

"Yeah," I said with a shaky voice, "I'll make it."

CHAPTER THREE

A Baby 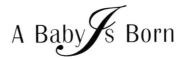 Is Born

August 22, 1993, 4:50 p.m.

Eric Zachary Thompson was born Sunday afternoon,
three hours after our arrival at the hospital. The delivery
was quick, easy, painless (after the epidural took effect!)
and, to some extent, not at all what I had expected. It was
quite low-key.

The team of doctors and nurses I anticipated did not
rush into my room. I was not lying flat on a gurney in a
sterile operating room with surgeons and an anesthesiologist
surrounding me all working intensely on my body's every
need. No nurse held my back up and screamed "PUSH" into
my ear as I sweated profusely from overexertion. No, I was
in what looked like a little girl's room: Pink flowered paper
covered each wall and the afternoon sunlight was shining in
one window, filtered by sheer nylon drapes. I covered myself
with flowered sheets and a pink blanket, snuggling into the
soft mattress of a twin bed.

Up until it was time to start the serious "work," there
were only three other people in the room: Patti, Bob and a
nurse who had also apparently done this a thousand times
before. Oh, and two brief visits from the doctor who was
going to perform the delivery.

"He won't come back until the baby has crowned," the nurse explained.

Once the monitor showed that my contractions were coming quicker and stronger, it was time for the start of the delivery. Patti sneaked out to wait in the lobby for my dad, taking the silenced tape deck with her!

"Bye, good luck," she said, grinning as she walked out.

At precisely 4:50 p.m. on August 22, 1993, I became a mother, acknowledged by the laughter, tears and life that filled the room.

Just an hour and a half later I saw Patti again, accompanied by my dad, Eric's grandpa. Bob had slipped out of sight for a moment to go and bring them in to see our precious, new baby boy. We exchanged warm and loving hugs as I held the baby close—all of us awed by this new life in our presence.

"He's so tiny," Patti said earnestly.

"He's only five pounds, six ounces, but he's healthy. He passed all the newborn tests and the doctor gave his thumbs up. Except for one minor thing, he's perfect! Look at his toes," I said, folding over the blanket covering his feet. "His fourth toe on each foot is raised a bit. The nurse said it's caused by a recessive gene. No big deal." I shrugged my shoulders and folded the blanket back over his feet.

It was time to move me into my room, and take the baby to the nursery. Bob packed up the few things I had used and we were off.

Starving, I said to Dad and Patti, as I finally settled in, "Would you guys go get us some food?"

"Sure. Where to?" Dad asked.

"Oh, I don't know, something hearty and delicious. Surprise me."

We spent the evening eating roasted chicken, drinking apple juice and celebrating our new life. Mark and Genie came by with Mark's mom, who was visiting from New York, to join the celebration. It was a remarkable evening. Love, joy and excitement filled our hearts—our spirits were high. Life was different now.

I just didn't know yet *how* different life had become.

CHAPTER FOUR

Down 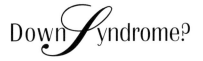yndrome?

August 23, 1993, 10 a.m.

The oatmeal they served for breakfast was cold and stiff —true hospital food. We kept the little four-ounce jars of apple juice and orange juice, and Bob went to the cafeteria for a couple of toasted bagels.

I was overwhelmed with a kind of joy that I'd never known before. My heart could have exploded from being overstuffed with love and excitement about being alive. The thrill of my life and my new baby's life kept me awake most of the night, my head swimming with the exhilaration of having a truly perfect life. Eric "looked like a little cherub" according to his cheerful daddy.

Thoughts passed like clouds blowing in the wind. My mind raced in all directions at once randomly reliving past events and envisioning events yet to come.

Just seven months ago I was standing on the busy corner of Pennsylvania Avenue and 14th Street in Washington, D.C. A cold January rain was chilling my bones while I waited for bus number thirty-two to come along and take me to my cozy home. My days were racked with frustration. The hour-and-a-half commute, the bitchy boss and temperatures that could frost even the warmest of hearts extinguished any flicker of contentment that ever arose during those two long years in D.C. As I stood on the east corner and watched my bus stop at the far corner—at which I was not—I lost all composure.

"This is it!" I exploded. "I've had it!"

I turned and marched the block to the 14th Street Station and took the metro to Union Station, where I bought a one-way ticket for the commuter rail home.

While I again waited, still grumbling "That's it, I'm done with D.C.," I telephoned home to let Bob in on my latest decision. "What's wrong?" he asked.

"I hate it here. I'm sick of this bullshit. I'm moving to Tampa. I can't take this one more day. I'm giving my notice tomorrow. I'm disgusted by this filthy city. I've got to get out of this place. I hate every day. I want sunshine and palm trees. Will you come with me?"

Ninety days later we were basking in Florida's sunshine!

Back further...

"Will you marry me?" he asked tenderly six years ago, embracing me. He was standing behind me, watching in the medicine cabinet mirror as I applied my mascara. We looked at each other's reflection. I was shocked. I wanted to scream "YES, YES, YES, I Love You! I've always loved you. Yes, I'll marry you." Instead, what came out of my mouth was "I'll have to think about it." *Who said that? You know you don't have to think about anything. You've always loved him. You've always known he was the one for you, just say YES.*

But, I don't know if he's really ready, I debated with

myself. *You know he's always had that one-day-at-a-time attitude. Why now? Just shut up and say yes. Okay, okay.*

Seconds later....

"I thought about it, and yes, I'll marry you."

Now forward...

I'm imagining Eric is about four, and the three of us are building a sand castle on Florida's Captiva Island. We're splashing water at each other and dumping sand on each other's feet. Laughter and love create the foundation for our castle.

Ahead...

Eric is four and picking tomatoes and zucchini and corn from Grandpa Ray's garden while Mom and I make dinner and chat about mom things.

Further forward...

Daddy and Eric take off early for a day at the ball park.

Eric hits a home run and is the MVP of the Little Leaguers.

Back to the present...

I was inundated with such thoughts. They kept coming,

faster than my mind could process them. I had been awake all night from the sheer joy of being alive. I was in love with my life, in love with my husband, and in love with my new baby.

Minutes later, Bob came back with the bagels, thank God. I was starving.

It was 10 a.m. and they hadn't brought the baby to the room yet. Odd, I thought. But he was premature—I guess they had things they needed to check out before we could see him this morning.

We were munching on our bagels when Mr. Magoo's look-alike came walking through the door. He introduced himself as Dr. Gage, the pediatrician. The new parents were beaming.

"I just came from seeing the baby," he said flatly.

"Oh," I replied, unconcerned.

"He's fine, there's just one problem."

With bagel in hand, my arm stopped dead in mid-air. All chewing ceased and I was left with a wad of half-chewed sesame-seed bagel in my mouth. My unblinking eyes were transfixed on this little brown man whom I didn't know. Years passed in this one moment.

"We think there's a chance he may have Down syndrome."

Trembling began in my fingers and traveled up my arms, down through my heart and into a twisted, churning stomach. My legs lay limp and numb. Sweat emanated from my feet and hands. My throat tightened as inhuman sounds came from it. My face contorted, pulled in one direction by terror and in the other direction by denial. Shock smeared away the smile leaving an opened mouth. My eyebrows pressed so tightly together that a pressure headache erupted. Unconsciously I dropped the bagel and spit what was in my mouth into a napkin. All desire for nourishment vanished.

The joy, that had just a second before filled my heart and pumped life through my veins, was oozing out of every pore. I was hollow, empty, scared, *shattered*.

"I don't want the baby," I cried. "I mean, I want a baby, my baby, but not this one. I want a normal baby. I don't want this baby." My hands covered my face. "I want a normal baby, I can't do this."

I finally looked up at Bob, my eyes begging for comfort, relief, waiting for him to somehow make it all better as he usually does. I'd never seen his face like that before. Tears welled in his bloodshot eyes, his face distorted. He was immobile. I saw no answers in those eyes where answers always lay. I knew instantly he could not "fix" this one, or make me feel better, or gloss over this moment with his timely wit.

I was alone, completely alone. There was nowhere to find comfort or peace. There was no way to change what this stranger had just said.

Could he be wrong? Yes, he could be wrong. He is wrong, I know it. This doesn't happen to me. He must have meant to tell the couple in the next room that their child is not normal. Our baby is normal. He is normal. I've seen him.

CHAPTER FIVE

The Social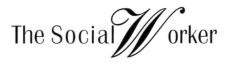orker

August 23, 1993, 10:45 a.m.

She waltzed into my room with a phony, nervous smile plastered on her face.

"Good morning," she sprightly said to two very distraught new parents. "My name is Tina, and I am your social worker."

"Social worker?" I questioned, upset, annoyed, wanting her to go away.

"Here is some information on Down syndrome," she said, handing me a cloth bag full of pamphlets. I was in shock, rigid, unable to fathom how she could be throwing these unwanted facts at me.

She pulled out a green brochure, opened it and handed it to me. "This explains what Down syndrome is..." she continued. But I had stopped listening. I looked down at the paper laying open in my lap and saw in big, bold letters **WHAT IS Down syndrome?** I had had a genetics class in high school and knew enough about this chromosomal defect that I didn't want any part of it. I couldn't move. My head remained bent over. I hadn't the will to look up. My gaze wandered to the passage below the title:

"Down syndrome... most common chromosomal abnormality in humans... only one that allows the embryo to develop... all races... all countries... one in one thousand births... 23 sets of chromosomes, one comes from the mother's egg; the other from the father's sperm... extra chromosome on the twenty-first... known as Trisomy 21... causes genetic imbalance... scientists do not know what causes... chromosomes stick together... forty-seven instead of forty-six..."

I slapped the brochure closed and tossed it on the bed toward the intruder. "I don't want to know this," I said in anger. I caught her off guard interrupting her Down syndrome parents *spiel.* I flung my hands to my face, covering my anguish. "I don't want this baby, I want my baby, I want my baby," I kept saying over and over again.

Her smile disappeared and her speaking shifted gears abruptly.

She told us we didn't have to keep him—our baby, our son, this little person for whom we've been waiting eight months, this little guy who waved to us from inside the womb during our six-month sonogram. On the monitor, he turned, faced us and waved hello. We learned during the same sonogram that Junior (temporary womb name) was indeed a boy. We were captivated, watching him roll back and forth, play with his toes, swim in the warm placental sea. Our hearts rolled and played along with him. He was a happy kid already and we were flooded with joy and fulfillment.

This is the person the social worker was talking about when she said we didn't have to keep him. "There are people who will take in babies like him when the parents can't cope," she told us.

Who the hell is this heartless woman who could tell a mother she didn't have to keep her baby? Didn't she learn

*compassion in some Social Working course? Didn't she know
we weren't thinking straight? How could she bring more sadness to where so much sadness already was? Who was this
woman?*

And I stopped.

Something in me shifted. Cruel though it may have
seemed, she was offering us a choice where no choice existed, where circumstances prevailed and forced us to somehow deal with this unforeseeable situation. I stopped
because I began considering this as a possibility. *We've only
known him eighteen hours—how long would it take us to forget? The sadness and despair could be gone, out of our lives
forever. We could, conceivably, hand over our baby to people
who claim they would take care of him. I trusted that to be
true, but could they hold him like a mother would, like I
would? Would they spend hours rocking him to sleep like I
would? Should we hand over our new rocker and the changing table and the few accessories that we did have, along
with our baby? Should we empty the nursery of all traces of
baby stuff and turn it back into an office? Should I secretly
slip a picture of myself into his bag of belongings in case he
ever wondered who his mother was?*

The social worker spoke hesitantly. "There was a couple
who had a baby about a year ago. The wife couldn't deal
with having a Down syndrome child, and they found out
about a woman in New England who would very willingly
take their baby." Her words seemed harsh, but I listened,
staring downward into nothingness, as she continued. "The
parents decided to give the baby up and paid for this woman
to fly down and get their daughter. After six weeks the parents' hearts grew weak. They wanted their baby back, so
they flew up north and got her." She spoke without judgment while my own thoughts continued. *Could I hand over*

the memories of the first flutter of life I felt, along with the diaper bag? Could I give away the loving, comforting kicks I remember so well, in a bag full of infant onesies? No, I realized, this wasn't a possibility for me. The young woman finished her social working and departed.

I knew I would keep him, but I didn't want to see the baby, not yet. My desire to nurse my newborn vanished. I needed to get out of the bed and away from this dungeon. I was being swallowed by despair. *This is not me. I'm not used to sadness.* I was suffocating. Thoughts of a now-twisted future tormented me. I needed to breathe again.

Dad slipped quietly into the room. There were no hellos or smiles exchanged. He simply walked up to my bedside and hugged me, holding me while I cried in his arms.

The nurse bolted through the doors interrupting my agony. "Do you want me to bring the baby in?" she asked.

"No!" I said wiping my face.

"Yes," whispered Bob, seated in the corner rocker.

My head whipped around to him. *Yes? Yes! He's dealing with it. He is going to "make it all better." Oh, how I loved him, his strength, his confidence, his ability to make any circumstance work out. He's a saint, a star, the love of my life. How lucky I am to have found him, my soulmate.*

I knew I was not yet even close to where he was, but I also knew that that simple word, "YES," he so quietly answered with would turn my life, our lives, around. Maybe sadness wouldn't loom over us — maybe things would really turn out okay. "Things always turn out," my grandmother, Meme, used to say. *Well, Meme,* I spoke silently into my heart, *could things really turn out this time? How I wish you were here to tell me so.*

"I'm going outside, Dad. Will you come with me?" I asked and he was already heading for the door, cigarettes in hand.

Dad hadn't seen the baby yet today, as far as I knew. I

had called him earlier, telling him about the baby. I was hysterical on the phone. He didn't react or get emotional or try to comfort me with shallow words; he just listened. And then he came. He's always been "here" for me, my strongest supporter, my closest friend and my worst critic all at the same time. He's always answered the phone when I needed him, and, once again, he was there for me. And now he's here, to walk with me, comfort me, support me and, in some way, help me find the reason for this tragedy.

I headed out the door—my first time in public as a new mother... of a Down syndrome baby. My scraggly hair was pulled back in a headband, showing off a pale, makeupless face with dark circles under my eyes. My sundress hung on me like an old dishrag as I stepped out into the world. My head and shoulders drooped from postpartum recovery and an unknown future.

CHAPTER SIX

Little 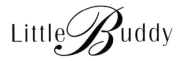uddy

August 23, 1993, 11:30 a.m.

"Thank God it was you," Dad said as we sat on the bench just outside the door of the hospital.

"What do you mean 'Thank God' How... how could you say that?" I asked, thinking he somehow wished this upon me.

"You can handle this. You have a loving relationship, you're full of fun and adventure. You laugh and enjoy life. You have always sought something different. Everything you've done is different than normal; this goes along with your life."

I listened intently, hanging on to his words, trying to sort it all out. "Who else signs up for the military at age sixteen, becomes a Russian linguist and moves to another country by age nineteen? You traveled the world looking for adventure; your twenties were incredible. You got married in Switzerland—what normal person does that? Eric is completely in line with how your life has been."

He was right and he was proud. I could see it clearly in his hazel eyes. I felt a release, slight though it may have been. I savored it, if only for a moment.

"Let's go back in," I suggested hesitantly. Bob was inside alone with the baby and I thought he might need us.

Dad nodded and grabbed my hand as we stood up. He put his arm around me as we entered that building, sensing my apprehension.

I opened the door to my room and the light shone through the window. The room was bright and clean. The bed was made and the uneaten food tray had been removed. Bob was standing near the window holding what looked like a rolled bundle of pale-colored baby blankets. He was singing softly gazing into the bundle. I could barely hear the song. It was *House at Pooh Corner.* I stared in wonder, surrendering to the melody.

Bob stopped singing.

"Hey, there, little buddy," he said through tears, looking up at me, "I'm keeping him. I've spent the last hour falling in love with him."

The denial and anger began to subside and I could sense a tinge of warmth and love start to seep in. I walked to Bob and looked down at the bundle. The baby's eyes were closed.

"Hey, Little Buddy," I whispered.

I kissed his cheek gently. "Little Buddy," I mouthed again.

"Can I hold him?" I asked fearfully, looking up at my husband.

"Sure," he whispered, smiling as he handed him over. I had never seen that loving smile on Bob's face before.

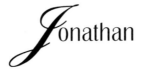 *J*onathan

August 23, 1993, 1 p.m.

I knew I had to call him and I was scared. What would he say? What would he make me do? No, not *make*, suggest; but it would feel like *make* just the same. I trusted him completely, though, and I knew what he would say would somehow, inexplicably, make what I was going through a little bit easier.

"We have to call Jonathan," I said, recalling the first conversation we had had with him about the baby nearly seven months ago. Although we had only known Jonathan for two years, our friendship seemed to transcend time. His forty years of life had been filled with a family of three siblings, an absent father, Vietnam, a contemplation of suicide, an engineering degree, a tennis coaching career, an extraordinary marriage and a project named "2000 LOVE." He began the "2000 LOVE" project in 1989 as a small tennis clinic to raise money for *The Hunger Project* and support its commitment to ending world hunger by the year 2000. The "small" clinic ended up being presented in the Capital Centre in Landover, Maryland in front of eleven thousand people and televised to more than ten million viewers. The players, who donated their time, included Andre Agassi, John McEnroe and Tim Mayotte. One and a half years after creating this project,

Jonathan accomplished the not-so-small feat of raising a hundred thousand dollars and stepped forward with a proud, yet modest smile when introduced as the Executive Director of the event. His five-foot-eight-inch frame stood tall as he acknowledged the guests, including the then First Lady Barbara Bush, with a slight nod of his head. His wondrous blue eyes showed a youthful soul that holds wisdom beyond its years. He was named ABC Evening News' Person of the Week, and graciously accepted an invitation from President Bush to visit the White House.

We met Jonathan just before he and his wife, Stacy, married in May of 1992. They had come up to us after a function and invited us to their wedding. They said they knew we didn't really know each other very well, but that they were inviting us for the friends we were going to be. They said they saw us in their future and thought they should act on it.

We eventually became the best of friends and, beyond that, Jonathan became sort of a "life coach" for us. He had spent quite a number of years in the training that deals in transformational technology, learning to free himself from his past, and to live life more powerfully and fully every moment. He had become somewhat of a master in helping others through conversation, to free themselves from whatever troubled them. The intensive coaching we received from him began about the time our new life came into being.

Seven months ago, after Bob and I had begun acting on our decision to move to Florida, we learned that I was pregnant. After three years of trying and a disappointing miscarriage, and in the midst of our excitement about moving, we were both disgruntled about the inconvenient timing and were very unsure about becoming parents. We made a dinner date with Jonathan and Stacy to work out our intentions for the move to Florida. That's not what we ended up talking about.

On a bitter cold and rainy evening, we met Jonathan and Stacy for dinner at a casual and fairly noisy restaurant. Jonathan was sick, coughing and sniffling as we were being seated at our table. He knew immediately something was *off* with us.

"Where are you guys?" he asked. "You're not here."

In the two weeks that we'd known about the pregnancy, we'd fluctuated between being thrilled and excited and upset and uncertain. We'd bickered over anything and spent most of the days preoccupied—going back and forth on whether or not having a baby was the right thing to do. At twenty-nine, I didn't feel ready. I had changed my mind, only it was too late. I knew Bob was concerned that I had changed my mind because he was, in fact, very ready. I told Jonathan and Stacy how the past two weeks had gone for us and how I felt about having a baby now. Bob sat quietly next to me.

"Why are you together?" Jonathan asked out of the blue.

Bob and I looked at each other, dumbfounded.

"What do you mean?" I asked.

"Why are you together?" he repeated.

"Because we love each other," I answered confidently.

"But what is the reason?"

"We have the same commitments, we both like to travel and have fun in life..." Bob was saying.

"I like his humor and his adventure," I interjected.

"We both want the same things out of life," Bob continued convincingly.

Jonathan stared at us. "But why are you together?"

"Because I want to be with him," I said, a little annoyed at his persistence.

"Exactly!" he exclaimed, perking up. "Because you say

so." He looked at Bob. "And you *choose* to be with *her*."

"Yes," Bob answered.

"When you get right down to it, it's all about choosing."

Without a word the waiter abruptly placed our meals in front of us. He apparently sensed the intensity of the conversation and rushed to leave our table.

"So, can you choose, really choose together, to have this baby?" Neither of us answered; there didn't seem to be a choice anymore. "Choose it as if you have a choice." He paused, then continued. "You know you can have it or not have it."

I saw tears welling in Bob's eyes. He was understanding what Jonathan was saying. He slowly turned to me and said, "We don't have to..." he hesitated, "We don't have to keep the baby." His words lowered to a faint whisper. "I know you're not ready." I watched the tears stream down his face and began to cry along with him. I knew how hard that was for him to say.

"We don't," I agreed, "and I don't feel ready. Even though I'm not ready, maybe the fact that I am pregnant means I am ready." I looked straight into his olive tinted eyes, forgetting that Jonathan and Stacy were across from us, and forgetting that we were surrounded by people eating, drinking and deep into their own conversations. I reached out for his hand. "Let's keep the baby," I said confidently.

"Are you sure?" he asked.

"I'm sure."

He wrapped his arms around me before another word was uttered and we hugged tightly. It felt like this was the first truly important life decision we had made together. It took our relationship to a level that was unknown to us just an hour before. We didn't realize it then, but that was to be the first of many life choices surrounding our baby and the first of many more levels to climb.

As we walked out of the restaurant, I heard Jonathan coughing. It occurred to me that he hadn't coughed or sneezed or sniffled during the entire conversation. He was so completely focused on us that even his own illness had been put on hold.

We were left alone in my hospital room. We had just spent an hour listening to our appointed pediatrician go on incessantly and aimlessly about "how special these types of kids are." Over and over he kept saying, "He's a special baby, he's a special baby. There's a lot these kids can do. Babies with Down syndrome are very lovable kids. You can love him like any other baby. These kids are special."

Special, special, special. Damn that word and damn him. How would he know anything about loving a Down syndrome baby? Who was he to comfort me? He doesn't even know me, us. He was an easy target, and beneath my shock and sadness lay a viciousness that secretly shot out at my unsuspecting victim. Emotions were uncontrollable and unstoppable. They had lives of their own, and could lash out at anyone without any warning.

Now we were left alone to somehow make sense of all that was happening. *How is this happening to us?* "We have to call Jonathan," I reiterated, the only sane words coming from my mouth.

"Okay, you call him," Bob answered sullenly, head bowed.

I sat cross-legged on the twin bed. The hospital gown fell from my shoulders, back opened toward the wall, tie undone. I hadn't bathed or even combed my hair since the delivery. I had neither the energy nor the wherewithal to pull myself together. Bob sat across from me in yesterday's wrinkled clothes, the same clothes he was wearing when he became a father. The black phone was between us near the edge of the bed. We had used it a lot already since the news came, and now it was time again. Scared and trembling, I watched my hand as it reached for the receiver and dialed.

"Hello," Jonathan answered cheerfully. *He answered. Damn. It's Monday morning, why is he home?* I wished he hadn't answered, I wished I hadn't called.

"Jonathan," my voice quivering, "It's Kim. The baby has Down syndrome." I blurted out. He silently waited for me to continue. "We don't know what to do... how to handle this. The doctor just told us. My baby is not normal, he's not normal. He said the nurses recognized a few signs during the night... something about creases in his left palm and his eyes slant a little. We didn't see any slant. They said they're reasonably sure, but he has to be seen by the Down's specialist, some Russian guy. All my tests were fine... I don't know how this happened. I wanted him to be as handsome as Bob. How could this happen to us?" I longed for some semblance of relief, grasping for a way to cope.

He spoke calmly, directly. "Have you ever had anyone close to you die?"

I was taken aback. The question seemed to be irrelevant. *Keep trusting,* I thought to myself.

"My Meme died three years ago," I answered tearfully.

"What was it like for you?" he questioned.

Still not knowing where he was going with these questions, I answered curiously. "I was sad and lonely and I missed her. I still miss her. She was my best friend after my parents divorced. I didn't know what life would be like without her."

"Did you grieve for her?"

"Yeah, I guess so."

"What you're going through right now is grief. You're grieving the loss or the death of the future you expected to have."

My tears dried as I listened, trying to understand his words.

"Tell me some things you expected with your baby," he suggested.

"He was supposed to look like Bob did when he was a baby, adorable with bleached blond hair... he was supposed to be smart and like to go to museums with me... play Little League... be popular and athletic in high school... get married... be successful... have kids..."

"You had his whole life planned out. Whether it happened that way or not, that is what you anticipated."

"Yeah," I answered sheepishly. I never would have thought I would have planned my baby's life.

"The instant women find out they're pregnant, their future alters and they unconsciously or consciously begin planning. You need to "complete" the future you expected to have so you can be free and open to anything that may happen. Your future looks unrecognizable now, doesn't it?"

I nodded, as if he could see me.

"And it's not good news. People are comfortable with their predictable futures. You and Bob need to sit down with someone who can listen purposefully to you guys relate everything about the future that you thought was going to happen. And everything about the baby that you think you shouldn't think or ever say out loud, even if you're ashamed. Don't let anything—*anything*—go unsaid. If it sounds horrible or mean, say it. Whatever you don't say will keep you from really being with and fully loving your son. Get someone who will listen committedly to you and not say anything in response to what you say. Tell him his job is to say: Is there anything else? and that's all. Don't let the person give you advice, agree with you or try to stop you from saying what you need to say. Make sure he knows right up front his only job is to listen."

I grabbed the breakfast napkin and a pen and scribbled "complete future." "Mark and Genie will do it with us. Mark even teaches a class called *The Power of Listening.* They'll do it," I said, regaining my energy.

"Great. Do it as soon as possible."

I could see the tension on Bob's forehead melt away and the tightness around his eyes and mouth loosen as he watched me and listened to the conversation. It was like looking into a mirror. I was unbelievably lighter, looking forward to completing my predicted future and slightly excited about having an unrecognizable one. The despair that I kept returning to began to dissipate, and I was becoming lighter.

"What else?" he asked.

I spoke without tears and less fearfully. "I called Raymond, my stepfather, this morning and he cried when I told him. Then my mother called me back crying and in minor hysterics. I don't want people to feel sorry for me. It feels like everyone will be sad every time they think of us or see us. My dad was quiet and acted differently, like he was okay with everything. That's not normal for him, but it was comforting for me. Also, Patti sounded upset when we told her." I wasn't sure where I was going with all this.

"You have to let people have their reactions. Everyone you know had a future planned for you in their own minds. Their reactions are a form of grief and fear, just like yours. Let them say what they need to say or be however they're being, and just understand that they're going through something also. People will use what they already know about themselves to cope, and others may try something new, like being quiet or okay with it all like your dad. Whatever they do, it's an automatic reaction, a mechanism, that they have no say about."

"I can see that." I could feel my heart mending, my body energizing, my mind quieting.

He continued for a moment, reemphasizing all that was just said. He knew I was getting it.

"Anything else?" he asked.

"No... yes, I'm sure there will be, but not right now."

"How are you doing?"

"Better, thank you. Like life may not be as horrible and terrifying as I envisioned."

He chuckled with relief as he told me his initial reaction when I had first called. It was funny: At first he wondered why I had called him and what he could possibly say that would make a difference. He told me that those thoughts flew by in a mere second until everything in life disappeared and he was completely with me, listening to every word. We sighed together and said good-bye.

Bob was eager to speak with him and to hear the full story of our conversation. I handed the phone over, laid back onto the pillow, closed my eyes and breathed.

A Broken 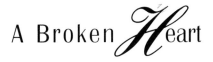eart

August 23, 1993, 6:30 p.m.

I hadn't held the baby since this morning, managing only a few glimpses through the nursery window. My body was weak from a lack of nourishment; not just sustenance, but the kind of nourishment only a baby's love can provide. I was drained and my head pounded from dehydration and sleeplessness. I couldn't cry anymore. In my weakened condition, I couldn't keep fighting off the anguish and feeling alone. I couldn't have been more heartbroken.

Dad had stayed with us all day, and Genie came by around dinnertime. We sat closely and spoke softly. Mostly, they listened while I continued to examine how this could have happened to me and how I was going to cope with this unexpected burden. Bob lay napping on the fold-out bed behind us. It was his first sleep since we were told about the baby.

Patti arrived at 7 p.m. her usual bright, bubbly self. I didn't understand how she could have such high spirits, and I resented her cheery attitude. Didn't she have any empathy for us?

"Hi!" she whispered jovially, trying not to wake Bob.

The room was dark again and wreaked of tragedy. Patti didn't know what she was walking into.

"What do you think of all this?" I asked ruefully.

"I just peeked into the nursery—he's beautiful!" she exclaimed.

She thinks he's beautiful? How could she think that? Doesn't she realize he's going to look like every other kid with Down syndrome? Wow, she really thinks he's beautiful! No one has said that yet.

"You know," she said, "I don't think this is so horrible. Bob said this morning on the phone that your lives were shattered. I've been hearing him saying that all day, over and over again in my head, and I just don't agree. I don't believe your lives are shattered."

I listened intently to her hopeful words.

"But it's not how we wanted this to go," I said.

"What ever is? That's the excitement of life!"

She was a godsend. For twelve years our friendship had flourished, and at that moment she was being everything I had always loved about her. Our friendship sustained the years in the military (she went to California while I stayed in Texas; she went to Greece while I went to Germany), six years of not seeing each other (communicating only through letters and cards) and two bad marriages (one for each of us). She was a huge influence in our decision to move to Florida. In her position as creative director for a major non-profit organization, she supported Bob in his determination to have a career in photography. After seeing his work, she not only hired him for every shoot, but also passed his name around town to her colleagues (she had seven years' worth of public relations connections in Tampa). She helped him fulfill a dream, and I got to be near my friend again. I had spent so much of the day in the dregs, I was ready to be pulled out. I knew I needed lots of help, and she was just the right person to provide it.

Patti's presence uplifted all of us. Our conversation turned to the opportunities available to us now that we had a baby with Down syndrome. We'd have to be different from anyway we'd ever been before... different... how do we change, though? What would I have to be like when people in the grocery store stared at my little boy? Or when kids at the playground didn't want to play with him because he wasn't like them? I was beginning to envision trips to the mall or the beach and ignoring all those stares. We could live in our own world made up of Mommy, Daddy and Baby, and to hell with everyone else.

"Or maybe," Patti was on a roll, "people would look at you and be inspired by the love you share." That was a stretch for me. She was going too fast, but I was opening up, breathing freely, ever so slightly.

"What if every look you got was because you're special?" Genie added playfully. That was certainly a different view than I'd been imagining. I was sorry Bob was missing this conversation, but he was resting so peacefully.

Suddenly, I had the urge to take a shower... clean up the room a little and let what was left of the daylight in. I was ready to hold the baby. Just as I stood up the door swung open and in walked a man in a white jacket with a stethoscope around his neck.

"Hello, I'm Dr. Johnson, the cardiologist."

"Cardiologist?" I questioned, glancing at my sleeping husband.

His expression never broke as he informed us of the baby's latest diagnosis.

"I've checked Eric out, and he has two holes in his heart." I dropped back into my chair." And a leaky valve. The small hole may eventually close, but he'll definitely need surgery to close the bigger one."

My head fell into my hands and I wept uncontrollably. He droned on in that same flat tone. The words melded together and I heard no more.

I was beginning to hyperventilate. Dad jumped up from his seat, came over and held me tightly. Genie knelt down in front of me, caressing my knee. I saw tears in her eyes and I could hear Dad trying to hold the tears in. I needed to know, but the question wouldn't come out. I tried again, caught my breath, and asked, "Is my baby going to...live?"

His answer sounded pitiless. "There's always a risk involved with open heart surgery. We can never guarantee success."

I doubled over. Dad was holding me now, crying with me. I know he was experiencing my pain, it's what parents do. I cried harder and harder. I wanted to die. I couldn't handle this; it was too much, too soon, too horrifying. Bob awoke and came over to me, hugging both me and Dad, begging us to tell him what was wrong. His cries were the last thing I remembered before everything blurred and faded.

CHAPTER NINE

Completing the 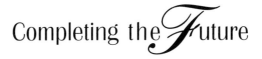uture

September 3, 1993

None of us knew what "completing on our expected future" meant, but we were willing to make it up as we went along. There were no rules. We shared a previous training course in ontology, the study of "being," so we had some common tools and distinctions to use for this process. We could allow ourselves to think anything and say anything — to cry, to laugh and to forgive ourselves in the end. We trusted that each of us knew it would all be okay.

We positioned ourselves comfortably around the living room: Genie on the floor cross-legged, Bob on the floor leaning back against the entertainment center, Mark sitting stretched out on the futon and me on the rocker, feet up on the couch. It was an intimate setting with a false calm blanketing our anxiousness.

The baby, only twelve days old, was already back in the hospital. The jaundice wouldn't go away, even after four days of intense ultraviolet light treatment at home. He was in for more intensive treatment and had to receive feedings through an N.G. (nasal-gastrostomy) tube. *My poor little baby.*

"What should we do?" Mark asked.

Remembering the conversation with Jonathan, I looked

at Mark and Genie and replied, "You are supposed to simply listen to us speak one at a time and ask if there's anything else to say. You're not to add or react to anything we say, and we should just say everything we've ever thought or expected or wished or dreamed about having a baby."

Having said that, my mind went completely blank and I had no idea what I needed or wanted to say. I was definitely nervous. "You start, Bob," I suggested, feeling a bit relieved.

"Okay." He seemed ready. I could see he was full of thoughts he believed he shouldn't be having. He started off with the good stuff, talking of wishes and dreams he had for the baby and the family. Fishing together, trying out for the *Baltimore Orioles*, things of that nature.

The afternoon dissolved as he talked. There was no time limit for this exercise; we were all there for the duration, until our future was complete and we could truthfully answer no to the question Is there anything else to say?

He would stop periodically, not wanting to say what was obviously on his mind. And then the prompt from Genie or Mark would come: "What else?" He'd jump that hurdle only to encounter the next. He delved deeper and deeper into his heart as he spoke of disappointments and fears.

An hour or two or three passed by. I sat silently as he spoke, relating to some things and getting upset over others, but always allowing him to say what needed to be said. After a while he wound down and, coming up with nothing more to say, he declared himself complete, although I knew in my heart there was something left unsaid, something so seemingly painful that it could not be verbalized. I didn't know what it was, but I knew it must surface before this night was over.

We stood up and stretched, refilled our water glasses and got more tissues. We changed positions and, once again settled in, all eyes fell on me. It was my turn. Mind still blank, throat constricted, palms sweating profusely, I took a deep breath and began.

I pulled from my past, recalling how sorry I felt walking into the middle of the school cafeteria and seeing the table of "special" kids eating lunch together. I remembered one boy in a wheelchair wearing a white helmet, and thought What kind of life will he have? is he having? I felt lucky.   There was one Down syndrome boy, too. He walked and talked like anyone else, but everyone knew on first sight that he wasn't the same as the rest of us. He would have to go through life with everyone knowing he was different, and to a pre-teen different was not good.

Those early opinions have stuck with me through the years. My fear of the "different" and my insistence on the "perfect" have kept me from even acknowledging the existence of anyone I considered "not normal." I would consciously turn my head if I saw a handicapped person on the street or in a mall, and I was never interested in watching television shows that depicted someone with a disability. I simply couldn't be with the "difference." And now I had to, and didn't know how. My thoughts were in conflict. I didn't want to look at my baby as though he were different, I wanted to accept and love him how he was. But those long ingrained thoughts fought hard to remain in place. I was confused. I didn't want pity, yet I pitied myself. *How would I ever learn?*

No one needed to prompt me to go on now. The more I talked, the more I had to say.

The perfect world I had created for myself had somehow turned upside down, and I was angry — angry at whoever or whatever in the universe gave me this child. I wanted to blame someone, something, but didn't know where to look. I sometimes blamed Bob because I asked him repeatedly to find out from his mother if his biological father had any "conditions" in his family. Since his father left before his birth, he has never had any connection to, or knowledge of, that part of his life. Late in my pregnancy, he finally asked, and his mom's answer was vague and uninformative: "I never heard of any problems."

Although her marriage to Bob's biological father was short-lived, I was hoping for more reassurance. Part of me wanted to undergo the extensive genetic testing to determine which one of us gave Eric his forty-seventh chromosome and, of course, it would have to have come from Bob since I was still living in my perfect reality. But once blame was determined, then what? I reconsidered and decided fault was not only irrelevant, but even destructive for our relationship.

"I'm sorry," I said to him.

"Thank you," he gently replied.

I was jealous, jealous of every friend who had a healthy baby. The jealousy spread to family members, co-workers, people walking on the street, the person next to me at a stoplight, even my parents. How lucky they and the rest of the world were to have healthy children. I resented watching parents yell or slap or ignore their children. Don't they know how fortunate they were that their children were healthy? Can't they see that children are a gift and should be nurtured and appreciated? I was the only one who ever had a handicapped child.

"How did this happen to me?" I asked pointedly, demanding an answer from my friends. They sat in silence as I waited for someone to tell me why. And then the answer came.

Mark asked, "Is there anything else you want to say?"

"Yes," I whimpered, "this is hard for me to say."

"Take your time," Genie said.

"I... I wish I had a normal baby."

Bob's tearful reaction told me he shared my feelings. I looked at him intensely, reading his eyes. I knew there was more for him to say.

After a few minutes of silence, Genie asked if I was complete.

"Yes," I said confidently, "but I don't think Bob is."

He wasn't. His face was contorted with repulsion, repulsion for himself, for thoughts that shouldn't occur and definitely not be spoken aloud, for thoughts that were choking his ability to speak freely.

"Say it," I said.

"I can't," he wept.

We waited patiently.

"Bob, we love you. Say what you need to say," Mark encouraged.

His mouth formed the words that were imbedded so deep in my own heart that my mind wouldn't acknowledge them.

"I thought... I wished he had died," he said. His head drooped with relief and disgust. I had had that thought, also, but lacked the courage to ever acknowledge it. We all cried for humanity and the courage it took to express such a thought, a thought that we knew we were not alone in having. Our future was complete. We were drained emotionally and physically. It was sometime in the early morning.

"Now what?" Bob asked.

"How are you doing?" Mark asked back.

"I feel lighter and a little empty. I feel like all there is for us to do is to love our little guy."

"I want to see him," I said. "I want him to know how

happy we are that he came into our lives. I want to hold him. Let's go to the hospital." I was rejuvenated.

The past was over and I was excited and eager to begin my future—my unexpected, unpredictable future—and I wanted to start it now!

I got up and went over to hug Mark. I thanked him for the valuable listening he gave to us and the safety he provided. I hugged and thanked Genie for her strength and determination that led us through that evening. They were truly remarkable, and a thank you and a hug could never show them the gratitude in my heart.

Bob and I hugged tightly and wiped our leftover tears away. We were stronger from this night and we were both ready for some love and fun again.

Genie and Mark opened the futon and snuggled into bed while Bob and I threw on our shoes. We drove to the hospital and spent the rest of the night beside Eric, our baby, loving him openly for what felt like the first time.

CHAPTER TEN

A Higher 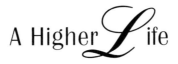ife

September 1993

In the lobby of a hotel, on the shore of Tampa Bay, I sat rigidly on the edge of the chair, my body stiff from an aching anger that tensed every muscle. My lips were pursed; my eyebrows strained to touch one another in a frown; my back was erect; and my feet set tightly together, were planted firmly on the floor. The chair was fluffy and overstuffed and, if one were so inclined, one could sink comfortably into it, hugged by its softness and warmth. But not me, not today. I glared at the bank of ordinary black pay phones hanging still and silent on the wall, barely noticing the blue morning sky through the window in front of me. The sun beamed into the room, warming my left shoulder.

I'm supposed to be in the room, I admitted to myself, *not sitting here waiting for the phones to ring.* I had volunteered four hours of my time to assist with this seminar that was taking place in a large meeting room of the hotel because Patti was in it, and I wanted to participate in the conversation that was going on in that room.

Even though the seminar was three days long, four hours was all I could commit because the baby was home and demanded constant attention. Bob and I took turns getting up during the night to feed Eric, who was still getting his formula through an N.G. tube that we had to carefully insert and remove with each feeding. His medicine schedule did not always match his feeding schedule, which added a couple more "wake-up calls" throughout the night. With the stress that came with being awakened every couple of hours, I couldn't leave Bob home alone with the baby for much more than four hours. Through the sleeplessness, irritability and constant fear that the baby's condition could worsen, we managed to work as a team, relieving each other when the stress became too intense.

Without any consideration for my situation or the obstacles I overcame in agreeing to volunteer, I was instructed to sit by the phones in case a call came in for one of the participants.

"For how long?" I asked the woman who gave me the instruction.

"I don't know, but we really need you out there. Please don't leave the lobby area."

"Fine," I said, storming down the hallway. *This is the last time I ever volunteer.*

Sitting, stewing, becoming more enraged, I looked around the room for something to read, or at least something interesting to look at. After a few moments, I began to notice how intense my emotions had become since the baby was born: Anger turned to rage, sadness to anguish and joy to jubilation. *Was this a normal, postpartum condition or was this a Down syndrome baby condition?* Simple disagreements with Bob would develop into fits of hysteria, leaving us both exhausted and upset. We would hardly ever arrive at a resolution; it was usually more of a surrender.

Unfamiliar emotions were ever present now, one of which was confusion about the baby's medical problems and how Down syndrome caused certain abnormalities. I didn't understand the severity of the heart defect, or the effect it had on his lungs.

Plus, I was overwhelmed by frustration when I nearly had to beg the health insurance company to get the necessary support. I was mortified that the insurance company had control over Eric's condition by denying or approving certain medical benefits. I realized how troublefree my life used to be. *Why did it take something like this to realize that?*

I wished for that time again. I had never seen anything but pride and happiness in other new mothers. *Will I ever feel that same pride and happiness?* My anger began to subside as my mind drifted aimlessly, thoughts about how life is and how it will be.

I snapped out of my contemplation as I glanced at my watch. It was 9:33 a.m., just three minutes since I had sat down. At 9:33 a.m. in the morning, I was already hoping I could catch a nap when I got home at 1:30 p.m., knowing that at the same time Bob would be in dire need of a Buddy break. I was tired, and succumbed easily to my own thoughts.

How could I have a baby with so many problems? No one in my family, as far back as anyone could remember, has ever had a Down syndrome baby. How could this have happened to me? Why? Will life ever be normal again?

"Hello!"

I was jolted from my thoughts and back into the lobby. I looked up in the direction of the friendly greeting.

"Hi," I said back to the stranger. He was not wearing a name tag, so I knew he was not in the seminar, nor was he volunteering for it. Who was this person who interrupted my solitude? I should have thanked him, but instead I was annoyed.

He must have seen the puzzlement in my face. "I'm sorry to bother you, my name is David." He sat down in the chair beside me, angling it toward me.

His face was pleasant, sort of young college professor-like, with brown-rimmed glasses and brown bangs brushed off to the side. He wore loose-fitting jeans with a nondescript, button-down shirt. With his hands resting on his knees, he leaned forward as though he were about to tell me a secret.

"I heard you just had a baby... a baby with Down syndrome." He spoke quietly, yet confidently, almost intimately.

Pushing myself back into my chair, I asked, "Who are you?"

"I'm Linda Sherry's boyfriend," he responded without movement. "You were in a seminar with her earlier this year."

"Oh, yes, I remember her." I eased up a bit, still wondering why he was talking to me.

"How's the baby doing?"

"He's okay. But, well, he has two holes in his heart that will need repairing through surgery, although we don't know when that will happen. The doctors say eight months to two years, but that Eric will let us know when it's time, whatever that means."

He sat listening intently, so I continued. "He had severe jaundice and had to go back into the hospital. They kept him for a few days under lights and began feeding him through an N.G. tube. Because of his heart problems, he's expending all his energy breathing, so he doesn't have any energy to eat. They told us to try to get him to drink from the bottle, but if he refuses or falls asleep, to feed him through the tube. We have nurses come to the house every day who have taught us how to insert the tube into his nose. Using a stethoscope, one of us has to listen for an air pop in his stomach while the other pumps a tiny bit of air into the tube with a syringe. My husband can do this alone now, but I still need help. The pop lets us know the tube is placed properly in his stomach and not in his lungs. If it were in his lungs and we fed him, he would aspirate. He also has laryngeal tracheal malacia, which means his larynx is loose, so when he breaths the larynx closes and obstructs his breathing. He has to crank his head back just so he can breath comfortably. The ear, nose and throat doctor talked to us about doing laser surgery, but he wanted to wait six weeks in hopes that the larynx will strengthen on its own. Other than that, I guess he's doing okay." My back rounded and my head drooped slightly. It seemed like so much.

I saw compassion in this stranger's face as silence settled between us.

"Do you know what exactly Down syndrome is?" he asked.

"I know that it's caused by having an extra chromosome on the twenty-first pair of chromosomes — instead of two there are three. And that third chromosome seems to cause random medical problems," I answered apprehensively, a bit bothered by his prying.

"Down syndrome is actually the result of mutated cells," he explained. "Mutated cells are the basis for evolution, and they're what lets species evolve. Down syndrome occurs across all races and has occurred continually over time. It doesn't seem to be stopping. It may never end. Just maybe, Down syndrome people are actually part of the evolution of human beings. Maybe they are a higher life form. Who knows?"

What's this man talking about, a higher life form? Could that be true? But if Downs people were a higher life form, why would they have so many medical problems? My mind paused while his words sunk deeper. *Maybe he means a higher life form in what is inside the body, in the soul, rather than the body itself.*

He continued. "They seem to have no judgment, and are full of unconditional love for people. They're always happy. What else is there? What else are people looking for besides love and happiness? If Down syndrome people do indeed have that love and happiness as a part of their being, their fundamental makeup, which seems to be true, then who's to say that they are not a higher life form? If they have what we're all after...."

He was abruptly interrupted by a quickly approaching figure. It was the woman who had sent me out here.

"You can go back into the room now," she said. "I'm replacing you here. You should go in right now, though."

"Okay, thanks," I answered as I stood.

I turned to my stranger-friend, looking into his eyes for an extended moment.

"Thank you."

Without breaking the gaze, he took my hand and held it firmly. "Congratulations," he said.

I watched him walk out the front door and into the sunshine. I never saw him again, but the possibility he expressed has stayed with me in my heart.

I hugged my replacement, turned and floated down the hall to the meeting room.

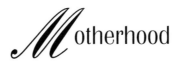otherhood

September 28, 1993

I hadn't seen my baby open his eyes for nearly two weeks. Eric was six weeks old and taking up residence in the ICU. Dehydration had put him back in the hospital originally, but during his second evening there, congestive heart failure coupled with collapsed lungs set off a Code Blue, which sent him to ICU immediately on a life support machine. He was being monitored around the clock, and we were there as much as our hearts could stand.

I caught a glimpse at the eyes in the mirror. They were penetrating. I turned to leave, but the eyes drew me back. They were sad eyes. The puffiness came from tearful days, and the redness and dark circles came from sleepless nights. The gaze slipped from the eyes to the image facing it. The face was blotchy red and slightly swollen. The scraggly hair hung shapelessly to the shoulders. The fragile body, still a bit fleshy in the abdomen area, drooped forward in defeat. The hands clutched the bathroom sink, desperately trying to keep the weak body upright. Grief had enveloped every thought again.

Where could I go to get away from this, she pleaded with the person in the mirror. *Will this ever stop? Will life be as great as it once was? How could it? How do I get through this? And once I'm through it, how do I go on? Life will never be as fun and exciting as it once was. It couldn't be.*

I looked beyond the eyes, back to the scene I had just left. He was lying there, so frail and helpless. His fragile, four-pound, thirteen-ounce body lay flat on its back, immobile. The medicines drugged him into a constant state of sleep and kept him completely paralyzed. I hadn't seen his eyes open for two and a half weeks, not even a flutter. I was not allowed to hold him and could only be with him during certain hours.

Tubes came out of him from everywhere. A wide blue hose ran from his little mouth to a breathing machine. A tiny clear tube spilled out of one teeny nostril. An IV dripped liquid into him through a needle that was tightly taped to his outer thigh. His ribs poked out from under a belt wrapped snugly around his chest to monitor his heart beat. White and black wires dangled from the belt. He had bruises on the inside of each arm and ankle, and needle marks on the side of his head. He was helpless lying there and I was helpless standing there.

The image in the mirror came back into focus. I purposefully stared long and hard into the eyes, searching for the happiness I used to see. Tears fell into the sink, blending with the drips from the faucet. I had waited so long to have a baby, never wanting to be strangled by the responsibilities or imprisoned by motherly duties. Once the choice was made, though, I was ready. It was another adventure, and I was ready for the joy and excitement a new life brings. And now this. I lowered my eyes. "What should I do, how can I remember this time in my life, this brief time in my life that I'm experiencing motherhood?" I asked myself.

"I have to write this down, all of it, my feelings, thoughts, fears, how it feels to touch his soft, baby skin, the love I feel when his big, brown eyes look at me, how truly comforting it is to rock him to sleep, everything." I said aloud looking into the mirror. And silently I said, "If I don't write it down and something happens, I may not remember, and I couldn't bear to ever forget...."

The 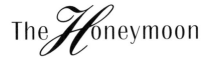oneymoon

October 4, 1993

We had missed their wedding. Tom, my father-in-law, and Sharon, his fiancee, had bought us airline tickets to California to make sure we attended. It meant so much to Tom that all four of his kids and their families be there to celebrate his special day with him. Even though Tom was not Bob's biological father, he had been his dad since birth, and Bob was his "first born." Tom was the only father Bob knew, and blood or no blood, Bob loved, respected and honored him, as did I. We wanted to go. We would have welcomed the change of scenery and an atmosphere of celebration. Bob almost went by himself, but Eric and I needed him more. His dad, though disappointed, understood.

So, Dad and Sharon changed their honeymoon plans: We were their honeymoon! They brought with them their wedding video, all the stories about the day's events and their love, and flew to Florida for five days.

We watched with excitement as they stepped off the ramp and through the arrival gate. Bob snapped a picture, catching bright smiles at their first sight of us. His dad whisked me up and twirled me around in his gorilla-like arms, laughing and hugging. He's a big man, six feet-two inches, with a booming voice that could scare anyone. But underneath is a very gentle, kind and loving man.

"How's my boy?" he asked Bob, smothering him with hugs.

"We're doing okay, but it's really great you came. Thanks for coming, Dad." They came to us because we couldn't go to them, and it was a time when being together meant more than anything else.

Our first stop was the hospital. They were eager to see their new grandson. They flew all the way from California to visit with him for a few minutes, kiss him on the cheek and hold his tiny hands. They knew on this visit there would be no rocking the baby, feeding him a bottle or playing patty-cake. It was the energy of their love he would receive on this visit.

"Hi, sweetheart," Sharon whispered in Eric's ear as Grandpa held his hand, "Grandma and Grandpa are here. We love you."

Their company was a breath of fresh air. It was like having a brief mental vacation. We showed them the town, ate snow crabs and Cajun shrimp, talked about relationships, living in Florida versus living in California, family and always, Eric.

We stopped to visit my mother in Ocala on the way to St. Augustine. It was to be a 24-hour respite in the oldest city in America. None of us had ever been there, but before we left Tampa, we made a stop at the hospital. This was to be the longest time we'd be apart from our little Buddy.

He had been intubated — put on a breathing machine — for almost three weeks. I could tell the doctors had gotten quite concerned by the second week when the pneumonia wasn't clearing. He was being given aerosol lung treatments every two hours followed by chest pounding with what Bob referred to as the "baby jack hammer." He was getting almost as much diuretics as he was formula to dry up his lungs. It was a battle to balance his liquid intake, with his liquid output. The foreboding that came with Eric teetering between life and death is what I woke up to every day. It was in the background of every conversation I had and what I went to sleep with every night.

Each day we'd go in and review his morning x-rays with the intensivist on duty. Some days the cloudiness on the x-ray in his lungs looked darker and other days lighter. No significant changes occurred the first two weeks until, suddenly one day, the lungs were almost completely clouded. "He's doing much better," the nurse had told us the day before. And now the doctor was explaining the possibilities and risks of performing open heart surgery on a sick baby. It wasn't a good option, but with this sudden turn for the worse, it may have been our only option.

His words threw me back into denial. I hadn't yet gone back to work from maternity leave and I waited daily to bring my baby home. I yearned to do all those motherly duties, something I never thought I was capable of feeling, or doing. My eight weeks of maternity leave had so far been spent primarily next to an ICU crib trying to be a new mommy. I felt like I was constantly fighting an uphill battle and I became numb. *What else?* I thought. *What more could go wrong?*

"Isn't he getting better? His lungs have been clearing, according to his x-rays," I argued.

"I understand. We thought he was doing better, too, but these slides prove his lungs are filling too quickly to wait very long."

67

The doctor explained the heart pumping process again—
we'd heard it at least twice before. "The large hole in the
ventricular area is causing the new blood and used blood to
mix. The heart is pumping the mixed blood into the lungs,
but the lungs are too weak to pump it out. The lungs get
overloaded, collapse and drowning could occur."

I interrupted. "I know why it's happening, but I don't
understand how he can be plummeting so rapidly when he's
been gradually getting better."

He had no answer for me. I could sense his commitment
was to saving babies, not to telling parents about down-
turns. He was only thirty-five, and he'd already dealt with so
many sick babies.

"Can you shoot another x-ray?" Bob asked hopefully.

"Yes," he said with some apprehension. "I'll call for
another before I contact the cardiologists. But you should
know if the second x-ray confirms his condition, you may
have to think quickly about scheduling him for emergency
heart surgery."

"Thank you," I answered, not really sure for what to be
thankful.

While we waited for the new set of x-rays to be read, we
told Eric about his grandparents from the West, that they
were coming to visit him soon and couldn't wait to hold him.
In between grandparent stories, we let him know that there
was a possibility he would need the heart surgery sooner
rather than later, and how unsettled we were about his
seemingly fluctuating health.

To mask the anxiousness, we returned back to the fun
grandparent stories and began to include other grandparents he had. It was apparent we had to distinguish for him
exactly how many grandparents he had and who they were.

"Well, let's see, " I said, getting ready to count them up

on my fingers. "Grandma Joan and Grandpa Ray are Mommy's mother and step-dad and live just two hours from us, as does Grandpa Jim, Mommy's dad. Grandpa Tom and Grandma Sharon are Daddy's dad and step-mom and they live in California. Grandma Rosie and Grandpa Dennis are Daddy's mom and step-dad and they also live in California. Grandma Francene is Daddy's ex-step-mom, but they're still very close. She lives in Oregon. Gram and Pop are Mommy's grandparents on my mother's side and they live in Philadelphia. Lastly, Peppe is mommy's grandfather on my dad's side and he's eighty-one years old. I think that is it; eleven in all! That's a lot of people who love you," I told him as he lay there paralyzed from medication and in a deep, sedated sleep.

Dr. Adams, the intensivist, returned from reading the new x-rays. He approached Eric's bedside with a wide grin across his face. He wasted no time in telling us the results. "*He is getting better!* It was a bad processing job by the technicians. I'm so sorry."

My eyes welled up instantly. Sad tears and happy tears were coming so frequently, I sometimes couldn't distinguish between the two. I was relieved he was getting better, on the other hand, I was still troubled because this so-called good news just delays the inevitable surgery. *Moment by moment,* I spoke firmly to myself, repeating it over and over again like a mantra.

Somewhere in the background I heard Bob's relieved voice rehashing the processing job of the old slides with the baby. Being a professional photographer, he understood how it could have happened. "You're getting better and that's all that matters," he whispered to Eric. "I love you."

69

Twenty-four hours in St. Augustine renewed our spirits. The four of us ate, went sightseeing, drank from the *Fountain of Youth,* laughed a lot, enjoyed putt-putt golf and played poker all night using cut-up pieces of paper for chips. Mostly, we shared each other's company, and that was the best part of it all.

We had to get back to Mom's by 2 p.m. for the baby shower she was throwing for us. The "star" guest wouldn't be appearing, but I brought pictures to show all the relatives who hadn't seen Eric yet. I just hoped I wouldn't notice any sadness in their eyes; I wanted to be strong for myself and for them, and I wanted them to be happy for me even in the midst of his situation. I needed their support and knew somehow their support would come from me.

We made it to Mom's house a half an hour early. Dad and Peppe were already there. Bob introduced all the parents and grandparents and began the tale of our trip to St. Augustine. Meanwhile, I darted to the phone to check in on the baby.

"He's stable," the nurse said. "Dr. Adams will be in to see him in an hour or two."

"Okay, if there's any change please call me at my mother's to let us know. Her number is at the top of Eric's chart."

The great-aunts and-uncles trickled in couple by couple until the living room, kitchen and patio were filled. Even though Eric couldn't be there, they were glad to see we were "holding up so well," as Aunt Rita put it, and they gave me extra long hugs. They all pitched in to give us $500 for the super-duper baby crib/toddler bed that I had been wanting.

This meant that he would grow to be a toddler; otherwise,

why would I get this bed?

After a couple of hours the party began winding down. Everyone had eaten all the food that Mom had prepared and barbecued, and quite a few had departed. Everyone who was left sat on the patio chit-chatting. The phone rang loudly from inside. I held my breath and looked up at Mom.

"I'll get it," she said, standing up.

A phone call these days could mean anything.

Mom came to the doorway and looked directly at me. "It's for you. It's the hospital."

Chills surged up my spine and my shoulders tensed. I wiped the sweat from my palms as I slowly arose. I stared at the telephone and walked toward it. With clammy hands, I picked up the receiver and quietly said hello.

"Dr. Adams just extubated Eric," the nurse announced.

"What does that mean? I don't know what extubated means." My voice quivered.

"He's off life support! He's doing wonderfully."

"Really, he's getting better?" I needed confirmation.

"Yes, he's been off for an hour now and seems to be holding his own. We're watching him closely, but he's looking good."

Adrenaline ran through my body, relieving the fearful tension and replacing it with excited tension. I sat down.

"Thank you," I said hanging up the phone. I sat for a moment, regaining any composure possible. I took a few deep breaths, stood up and headed toward the patio. I stopped at the doorway and just looked at everyone. There was dead silence as they stared at me, awaiting the news.

"They took him off life support. He's doing better," I said smiling, joy filling my heart.

I saw the relief pour out of everyone's eyes before I was engulfed in Bob's embrace. This scare was over.

Home Away from *H*ome, Part I

August - December 1993

- Aug 24   Eric and I were discharged
- Aug 26–31   Eric had in-home light treatments for jaundice, sixteen hours each day with daily visits from home health nurses
- Sep 5   Eric was admitted for failure to thrive and a high bilirubin (extended jaundice) count
- Sep 10   Eric was discharged
- Sep 15   Eric was admitted with dehydration and respiratory distress. Just days after admission, Eric suffered from congestive heart failure and collapsed lungs. He was put on life support for nearly four weeks. After extubation (taking him off life support), a hearing test was performed in which they determined he was deaf, (this turned out to be not true)
- Oct 29   Eric was discharged on constant oxygen
- Nov 10   Oxygen was discontinued
- Nov 22   Oxygen was prescribed again

- Dec 6   Eric was admitted with pneumonia
           (my thirtieth birthday)
- Dec 10   Eric was discharged
- Dec 17–21
           Eric was admitted to the hospital
           with pneumonia
- Dec 27   Eric was admitted to the hospital
           with pneumonia and heart congestion

Christmas in Seattle, 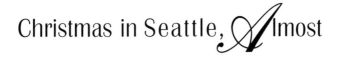lmost

December 24, 1993: One hour before departure...

Bob stood, eyes lowered, holding the receiver to his ear. His head drooped as he shook it from side to side as if beaten, surrendering. I knew at that moment we weren't going.

Our insurance company had cut Eric down to four hours a day of home health care. His nurse, Tracy, just twenty-three with long blond curls, was sitting on the floor next to him listening pensively to the phone conversation. She was giving Eric his aerosol treatment while he lay on his tummy, strapped loosely into his styrofoam wedge. The position enabled him to push up with his arms and turn his head away from the light stream of mist. Tracy was more persistent than he was, though, and followed his nodding head to keep the flow of medicine directed toward his nose and mouth.

He had been out of the hospital only three days; another bout with pneumonia—his fourth in four months of life. *How long could his little system keep resisting?* The nurses were coming every day since his discharge to help him fight off the wetness that so regularly filled his lungs.

For two months we had been planning to use the airline tickets Bob's dad sent us earlier this year (originally to attend his wedding in California) so we could spend our first

Christmas with his side of the family in a suburb of Seattle. We both loved the Seattle area. The fir-lined, cobblestone streets reminded us of Germany. I was desperate for a change of scenery, refreshing conversation and to be around new people who weren't clothed in white coats.

Night after night, I busied myself in our 800-square-foot apartment attending to Eric's needs, while Bob was out playing acoustic guitar gigs, trying in the midst of our circumstances to keep his dream alive. His drive was immeasurable. I respected that, and it seemed any forward movement in his dream was the only source of excitement either of us had. Despite my support and enthusiasm, leaving up to four nights a week at six, seven, or eight p.m. to go to a gig didn't fare well with me, and we often argued before he went out for the evening. Eventually the anger would subside, and I usually spent the rest of the evening regretting my outburst. If I could stay awake, I would wait up for him to come home so that I could apologize. If I was asleep, he would tip toe in and apologize with a warm hug. The strain on both of us was immense, and sometimes screaming at each other was the only form of release available. Thank goodness our relationship was solid enough to sustain such a beating.

I didn't resent him for being out at bars and restaurants at night. His dream to make it in the music business was for *our* future, and I knew that. It was singing his heart out every night that had me gritting my teeth as he walked out the door; I could not find an opportunity for the sweet release of stress and emotions that I also craved. I wanted to run as fast as I could for miles and miles or yell until I had no voice left. Instead, I stored my emotions inside my body until I found a few minutes of nothing to do. I savored those moments of nothingness and sat quietly, motionless, breathing deeply, letting go... until a whimper and soft stirring sounded from the cradle.

It would be time to attend to the baby again. I understood this attention was no different than for any other new mother except that Eric lacked the energy to cry out when he was hungry or move when he was uncomfortable. His energy was used up by his body for breathing. Sucking a bottle was simply out of the question. I poured Eric's formula into a plastic bag that hung from an electric feeding pump. I wound the long, clear feeding tube around gadgets on the pump—reminding me of threading the sewing machine I never used anymore—and connected it to a one-inch tube that protruded from my baby's stomach. While the pump fed Eric over a one-hour span, I measured the 7 p.m., 10 p.m., 2 a.m., and 8 a.m. medications and set up two more bags of formula for the nighttime feedings. Bob would be home around midnight to start the first night feeding. We welcomed and quickly fell into the security and safety of a routine whenever Eric was home.

Bob pulled the receiver from his mouth and looked over at me, "Sharon's three-year-old grandson in Seattle is sick," he groaned.

I thought back to the excessive number of work hours I used up on the telephone contacting Eric's doctors—the intensivist, the cardiologist, the pulmonologist, the gastroenterologist and his pediatrician—getting their okay and any instructions for us to take the Seattle trip. I also coordinated with the airline to prepare oxygen during the flight and to have an attendant on the ground waiting for us in Memphis with an oxygen tank during the two-hour layover. On top of all this, we had to pay an extra $600 for this special care.

There was a hospital near Sharon's daughter's house where we would have to take Eric if anything were to happen. We were well prepared, we thought.

I labored daily over the decision to go ahead with the plan. *What would happen if the pneumonia recurred?* We would have to stay out there. *What if our insurance company wouldn't pay for the stay? How could we miss more work than we already had?* The thoughts lingered. On the other hand, Bob's parents were extremely excited to see their grandson, and Bob hadn't spent Christmas with his family in over ten years. I was compelled to take the risk. Until this.

"Forget it," I said. "It's not worth it. We'd be afraid the whole trip." I looked at Tracy, and her expression showed she agreed with me. Bob knew it, too, of course. I saw the disappointment in his eyes, mixed with the realization that we must keep our baby in as healthy an atmosphere as possible. A lump came to my throat, but I resisted the tears this time. There would be other trips and visits when Eric would be healthy. At this point, helping Eric avoid sickness and gain strength was more important than anything else in our lives.

Bob chatted for quite a while, consoling his dad's disappointment as well as his own while I began planning alternate Christmas plans, the two-hour road trip to my mom's home in Ocala. We had spent many weekends there with and without Eric in the past few months trying to escape, cope and rejuvenate, and we'd spend Eric's first Christmas there, as well.

Ten minutes later...

"Mom, it's me. How would you like company for Christmas?" I asked knowing that she would love to have us.

"Of course!" she answered excitedly, then added with a slight shift of tone, "What happened?"

I told her briefly about the series of last minute complications and the final decision that changed it all. We quickly changed the subject to what we would make for Christmas dinner and who to invite. Mothers are so wonderful; I felt better already. Mom had saved us so many times, when we just couldn't do it anymore. We'd go to her house in the country, a place where time stood still, where we could escape to a night of rest. We'd pack up the baby, the oxygen tank, his monitors, formula and some toys and unpack them in his room at mom's. She would hold him in her loving arms all evening while we relaxed and she would wake up early with him, letting us sleep in.

We hurriedly unpacked a few non-essentials, previously destined for Seattle, and were on our way.

Christmas morning was a brisk fifty degrees, not uncommon for winter in north central Florida. The celebration began early, 6:30 a.m., and although Eric didn't yet know about Santa Claus and wasn't yet eager to open all of the presents he had under the tree, he still woke promptly before dawn squirming for "breakfast." Bob set up his feeding while Mom fixed breakfast for the rest of us.

Meanwhile, I unwrapped Gram's present for Eric knowing it was a baby Santa suit. Even if Buddy didn't know what was happening, the love and joy of having him home with us at Christmas seeped into all our hearts, and fun and laughter filled the day.

After my dad arrived, we dressed Eric in his new suit and Bob proceeded to shoot off a roll of film. We hid the gastrostomy tube underneath the clothes, but there was no hiding the oxygen canula. I put the Santa hat on his head while Dad propped him against the pillows in front of the tree.

Mom and Raymond stood behind the camera making silly grandparent gestures, trying to get Eric to smile.

"Let go of him so I can shoot," Bob said to me, giggling over the sight of our elfish son. "Okay... ready... shoot." Just as I let go, he began to tip over. Dad caught him just as the flash went off! As the pictures showed, Dad's hand was shot stretched toward the baby in a "catch" position. We clapped after each snap and laughed and played together all morning like a bunch of five-year-olds after opening their toys, only our toy was Eric.

I guess the doctor was right, after all: He is a special baby. This special baby has brought so much love into so many hearts and closeness into so many estranged lives. How could I have been so afraid to have such a special baby?

CHAPTER FIFTEEN

Living with 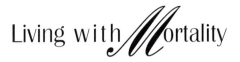ortality

December 1993

I walked into the house, stopping abruptly, in front of
Bob, who was standing in the kitchen doing the dishes. I
glanced beyond him into the dining room at Jonathan, then
drooped my head, the tears came immediately. I became
inconsolable. I wept into Bob's chest as he held me tightly. I
had just come from my Wednesday night yoga class, which
is normally a time of the week when I relax and stretch and
arrive home feeling refreshed and rejuvenated. Not this time.

At the end of each yoga session we always spent twenty
minutes resting in *svasana*, a relaxation pose practiced lying
flat on the back, arms and legs comfortably out to the sides
and palms facing up. This position calms the muscles after
a strenuous session and calms the mind after a stressful
day. This particular night, the teacher, an older woman in
her late fifties who healed her crippled body through fourteen years of yoga, instructed us to gently assume the
"corpse" position.

I had heard *svasana* referred to as the corpse position
only a few times since I had begun yoga seven years ago.
Something about her deep, somber voice saying "corpse" res-
onated throughout my body. I kept hearing her say, "corpse,
corpse" over and over again in my head, and then the words

turned to "death, death, dead, dead, he's dead, he's dead." I
wept in silence as I lay there thinking about Eric back in
that same icy, steel crib in the ICU. Pneumonia again. His
fragile little body didn't have the strength to fight off the
virus that so persistently attacked his body. *How much
longer could he take this?*

After three weeks without the oxygen in November, the
pneumonia returned suddenly one night. We rushed him to
the emergency room at 4 a.m.; I had been kneeling beside
his cradle for hours, rocking it, and when that didn't soothe
him, I held him close, patting his back while rocking my
own body back and forth. My knees and thighs ached, my
arms were weary, my spirit was drained and still his coughing persisted. I knew it was time once again for the emergency room. That meant the rest of the night and into the
morning dozing in the rocking chair, holding the baby (hopefully), if he wasn't too sick, in the pediatric emergency room
until a bed was ready for him in ICU. Then there would be
no rocking the baby in the days following.

"Don't be sick again," I pleaded with him. "Please,
please, get stronger. Be healthy," I whispered into his ear.

Bob got out of bed and began dressing. He too knew the
virus had won again. He took the baby from my arms while I
dressed. Within minutes we were out the door.

Six days later he was back home along with twenty-four-
hour nursing. In just another four days he returned to the
hospital. Midnight runs to the hospital were becoming
usual.

A couple of months back, Bob began taping an update of
Eric's condition on the answering machine, so callers could
find out how Eric was doing since we were often unreach-
able and the use of cell phones was not allowed in ICU.

I had spoken with Dad over the phone after Eric was

readmitted. There was something he had wanted to say to me, but couldn't seem to get the words out. He was unusually quiet as I related to him Eric's continuing health problems with this latest admission to the hospital.

"I want to say something to you, but I'm not sure how to say it," he interrupted.

"What?" I asked, noting his serious tone.

"Maybe, maybe..."

"Maybe what?" I asked desperately.

"Maybe, it would be for the best if he didn't make it."

Jarred by his words, I sank back in the chair. The thought was hauntingly familiar. Hopelessness had also touched me, but somewhere along the way I had realized I wasn't willing to give up.

"I just had to say it," he said. "For you."

"I understand, I've had the same thought, but... not yet, Dad, not yet."

Following this relapse, Dr. Mazor's office called. I was busy at the computer reconciling November's checking account balance when the phone rang.

"Hello." I spoke quietly, as Bob was napping on the couch.

"This is Dr. Mazor's office calling. Could you hold please?" a woman's voice asked.

"Hold? " I thought. "You called me!" *Why would they be calling me? It's been four months since the delivery.* I hung the phone up abruptly — go away — strangely shaken by this unexpected, unwanted call.

The phone rang again.

"Hello," I answered, annoyed.

The same voice repeated the greeting.

"That was rude to call me and put me on hold," I said. She apologized and, in the same breath, informed me that abnormal cells had appeared on my recent Pap smear. And would I like to make an appointment to see the doctor again?

"Oh, my God," my voice shook in fear. "What does that mean?"

The receptionist was obviously the wrong person to ask, so I made an appointment and asked her to page the doctor immediately. The earliest appointment opening was in January, almost three weeks away.

"What's going on?" Bob asked, still holding me after I broke down upon return from yoga class. I couldn't answer. It was death lingering so close that shook my insides. With the baby in the hospital again and my biopsy in two weeks, the word "corpse" had penetrated too deeply.

"Do you want to talk?" I heard coming from the dining room. It was Jonathan. *How is it that he answers the phone at the right moment, that he's here at the right time, and that he and Stacy choose to move to Florida to revive his tennis coaching career and kick off her writing career... all at the right time?*

I sat at the table across from him and told him what had triggered this reaction: the "corpse" occurrence, my test results and Eric's constant fight for life. He listened to me so intently; it was like nothing else existed for him. For two hours we went back and forth.

"What does death look like to you?" he asked.

I envisioned the world without me in it, and for me the

only thought that came up was "lonely." I would be alone.

"What would it be like if Eric were to die?" I was frightened by the question and hated him for stepping over that boundary. *How could he ask me that? Doesn't he realize it's not something I talk about?*

He asked again. I couldn't answer. I thought if I acknowledged his question it would somehow make it happen.

He asked again.

"I can't answer, I can't think it, I don't want to talk anymore!" I cried.

He waited, allowing me to calm down.

"It would be lonely," I whimpered " I don't want to live without him."

"Do you think Eric would feel alone?"

"Yes, of course," I answered.

"Eric is four months old. Do you think he knows the concept of aloneness?"

"Well, no, how could he? It's me who feels that he would be alone, or that I would."

"Exactly. Can you see that maybe you perceive death as loneliness, or aloneness?" I nodded. "Are you comfortable being alone?"

"I think so," I said. "Mostly when I am alone I'm doing something like reading, writing or exercising."

"Everything, but be alone with yourself," he said. "You meditate, don't you?"

"Yes, but not much lately."

"Maybe that's what there is for you to do now, consistently. Use meditation to explore the thoughts and feelings that are revealed around the subjects of being alone and with death."

My thoughts drifted back to Eric, alone in the hospital.

Does he feel alone, or is it just me feeling alone for him? Does he sense loneliness, or is that something learned as a person grows? Does he know how often he'd faced Death since his birth, or is it just me assuming he knows. Is he afraid, or is it me who is afraid—and so attached to my fears that I'm even afraid to let them go? As the conversation continued, a sense of peace replaced the foreboding, and I relaxed, allowing me to ponder these yet unanswered questions.

"Thank you," I said as I reached across the table and grabbed hold of his hands. "Can we talk more about this in a month or two?"

"Of course," he said endearingly. "Anytime."

In the next six weeks, I saw the doctor and got the results of my tests back. "Level one dysplesia," he called it. I went through a minor, in-office surgery which, I was told, "wiped out the bad cells."

In the same six weeks, Buddy returned to the hospital again with pneumonia. Once that cleared up, he went through a cardiac catheterization, so the doctors could look at his heart more closely to see if it was time to do the heart surgery.

"He's not ready yet," the doctors told us.

CHAPTER SIXTEEN

Another 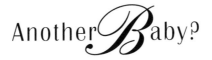aby?

March 1994

Occasionally, friends or family would dare to ask me the unanswerable question: Would I have another baby? It's a liberty they would take, probing deeper than an everyday "How are you doing? How's the baby?" question. They were aware at some level what I've been through emotionally. It may be a typical question asked of a mother of a healthy baby, but not usually accompanied by that serious undertone and look of concern.

I didn't know how to answer, so, consequently, my answer changed almost as frequently as the question was asked. I occasionally even asked myself *Can I go through nine months without worrying about whether the baby will be born healthy? No!* I'd reply one day. I hadn't reached a point where it didn't matter. The next time my answer would be *Of course! I'm stronger now.* Then, *one baby is all we ever wanted.*

Geared up for an evening of laughter and fun while driving with two friends to the comedy club where another friend was debuting as the emcee, the question arose once again. My good friend Gloria, a forever childless woman who chose to spend her life free from the gender struggle that occurs in any heterosexual relationship, posed the question after inquiring about Eric's health.

"So, do you think you'll have another kid? Sandy said she wanted to have another, but was afraid because she thought no baby could be as great as Benjamin."

Sandy, whose age fell into that danger range where an amniocentesis was advised, had given birth to a healthy boy just one week after Eric was born. I couldn't bring myself to go to her baby shower, which took place at the hospital the day after Benjamin was born since he, too, arrived a month early. The envy I felt every time her or her baby's name was brought up remained lodged deep inside, but would emerge when I was alone. The resentfulness quickly turned into disappointment. I just couldn't see her, it was too soon. It took me a year to finally meet her baby on his first birthday.

"What do you think?" Gloria asked again about having another baby. I was lost for a moment, wondering how to answer.

"No... not... not... well... no... maybe..." I was interrupted by their laughter. "I guess I'm not sure," I finally replied, joining in with their laughter and realizing how silly I must have sounded.

"I guess you're not sure," Gloria agreed.

"Every time I think about it, I come to a different conclusion. I've thought about adopting a three-year-old girl, later, after Buddy has been healthy for a year or two. If we were to adopt, at least I'd know she was healthy. Also, she would be close to Buddy's age— he'd have a playmate and she'd be out of the diaper stage."

They listened, allowing me to speak my thoughts aloud.

"Bob says he doesn't want to have another baby, adopted or not. He said Buddy fulfills all his fatherly needs. I think it's just too soon for either of us to make any decisions."

I heard sighs of agreement from my companions.

"Soon after Eric was born I wanted to get pregnant again right away. I don't think I could have handled being pregnant at the same time Eric was always in the hospital, but it seemed the thing to want. A couple of parents I met through *Up with Downs* had had a second baby right away, and it was great for them. Both of their next two children were born perfectly healthy."

I kept going. "But just a few months ago, my dad was in the post office and saw a woman with two Down syndrome boys. He introduced himself to her and told her his grandchild was also Down's. She told him both boys were hers and that she'd had them a year apart. Figure those odds."

Taking a deep breath, I continued. "The woman who owned the night school where I taught computer classes last year used to work with Down syndrome kids and children who were born deaf and blind because their mothers had measles during pregnancy. Wow, that would be hard. Anyway, first she advised me to keep my relationship with my husband intact and not worry about more children. "Concentrate on your marriage. It's the most important thing," she said. Then she sort of said I owed it to myself to have a "normal" child. I guess everyone has an opinion about situations like mine?"

"Interesting," Gloria replied under her breath.

"Bob and I were at the beach with my dad a few months ago and saw a family of four playing and splashing each other in the ocean. There was a little girl, maybe three years old, and a blond boy about five. He was jumping on his dad's back and the dad would swim around with the son on his back until the son fell off. They laughed together. I noticed that when I saw the family I felt happiness, but it abruptly twisted into sorrow. Buddy was in the hospital, and

I wondered if I'll ever be able to play in the ocean with my son."

"Why did you think that?" Gloria asked.

"Because Eric has been sick so much and he's so susceptible to illnesses. It's hard to tell how healthy he'll be when he gets older. Although, the nurses at his day care center said the first two years were the worst medically and he'll eventually get stronger and healthier.

"Anyway, I couldn't keep my eyes off the family. I kept hoping my future would look like that. After hard playing for quite a while, they walked up on shore together and I couldn't believe what I saw."

"What was it?" Dorothy asked while keeping her eyes on the road and her hands on the wheel.

"The little boy was Downs!"

"That's great!" Gloria cried.

"It was so *great* to see," I agreed. "So, about having another kid, I don't know. Ask me again next year if I don't yet have another baby."

CHAPTER SEVENTEEN

Our First 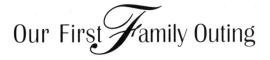 Family Outing

July 1994

Eleven months and two days after Eric was born we had our first official family outing. We'd gone to Grandma's for the weekends, popped into the grocery store and barbecued at the Clark's home occasionally, but that Saturday was our first day out together. All three of us. Just to play and have fun together.

It started off like many previous Saturday mornings. Eric awoke wide-eyed at the crack of dawn and woke me up with his morning gurgles of hunger. His early morning formula feeding had kicked off around 5:30 a.m., so he was hungry for some solid food. In my half-awake state, I fed him oatmeal with apples and bananas while Bob graciously made coffee and whipped up banana waffles sprinkled with blueberries for us.

As we enjoyed our delicious breakfast, we began planning what to do that day. We planned to take turns being with the baby and doing whatever it was each of us wanted to do for ourselves in between, be it running, reading or just relaxing. Even though medically the baby didn't need quite as much attention as he once did, he demanded at least one of as a playmate, or companion most of the time. After weeks of wondering whether he was going to live or die, I never resisted his desire for me to play with him.

After all the chores of the day were laid out, Bob said excitedly, "Let's go to the zoo!"

I got excited, too, but immediately became concerned. "What about the heat and the feeding?" At fourteen pounds and still on a liter of constant oxygen, there were things to consider when taking him out, especially this first time.

"We'll just pack the twenty-ounce syringe and feed him in the air- conditioned snack bar," Bob answered, still excited at the prospect of going out together.

Eric had been doing so well for a couple of months, and now with the small tank of liquid oxygen we were much more mobile. I couldn't resist. "Okay, let's go! But let's go buy one of those lightweight strollers so he can sit upright. That carriage is too small for him now."

It was a beautiful, sunny summer morning and we were going off to have our first family day together. We were beside ourselves with joy. During my last six months of pregnancy, we had strolled through the zoo talking about the day we would bring our baby here, wondering which he would like the best, the pink flamingos, the graceful manatees, or perhaps the playful baby orangutans. Going to the zoo had always been one of our favorite ways to spend a relaxing day together. We had hit almost every major zoo in Germany when we lived there and now we couldn't wait to share the zoo with our son.

Daddy and Eric, sunglasses donned and smiling at the camera, posed at the entrance. Snap! We proudly walked through the entrance gates together.

Our first stop was the water fountains, where we cooled

off before heading into the park's maze. As I held Eric near one of the spouts, kids weaved around us, jumping over the spurting water, running and laughing as they got wet. In the hubbub of the playing I noticed a boy with Down syndrome about four years old, giggling and drenched like everyone else. I stared a moment; it was like glimpsing into our future. *Someday when Eric is a littler older and stronger, he and I will run through this fountain laughing and playing and getting soaked together.* Meanwhile, I was conscious of his oxygen and careful not to get water in his ears because of the tubes. I held him tightly as I splashed water on his tummy, arms and legs.

The day was glorious! Eric was mesmerized by the waterfall at the monkey site, but didn't care much about the monkeys themselves. He liked the trees, the cool breezes and the other kids being pushed in their strollers. We pointed out the ruby-red baby spoonbills and told him about alligators. We sat in the dimly lit, air-conditioned room in front of the water tank watching a manatee swim by nudging at his iceberg lettuce lunch. His eyes followed the otters as they twirled and whirled underwater looking like they were having so much fun just being otters and doing otter things. *How delightful it must be to be an otter,* I thought!

We stopped to feed Eric at the snack bar. He gobbled down mashed bananas and flirted with the little girl at the next table. He smiled and she smiled and then her parents smiled and we smiled—what joy babies bring to everyone.

Eric and I hung out on the walkway between the turkey and the deer sites while Daddy went to get us a bottle of water. Eric drank apple juice from his bottle, holding it himself with both hands. After not having the mere energy to suck from a bottle for so long, it was thrilling to watch his big eyes peering over the top of the bottle at me as he sucked and sucked, apple juice dripping down his chin.

As we waited, I enjoyed eavesdropping on the conversation next to me. Speaking to a disinterested one-year-old, a dad asked, "Do you know how turkeys talk? They say gobble, gobble, gobble." On the other side of me a mother was gobbling at her son until he finally ran off. Across the walkway, the kids were yelling excitedly about seeing Bambi, a fawn lying next to its mother.

The outing was nearly over, and as I drove home, Daddy and Eric slept peacefully after a big day at the zoo. I smiled as I thought *Could life be any better than today? Maybe this is, in fact, what life is all about: loving and playing together.*

CHAPTER EIGHTEEN

A Moment to 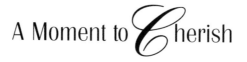herish

November 1994

I peeked at my sweet little boy from behind the kitchen
door as I stood at the counter chopping vegetables for a stir-
fry. He was completely preoccupied with struggling to pull
himself to a standing position. I watched his palm-sized
behind rise up in the air, performing a perfect Hatha Yoga
"downward dog" posture—legs straight, hip-width apart,
heels on the ground, sacrum reaching upward, body bent
over, hands firmly planted on the ground, fingers spread
widely open, arms straight and head relaxed! Unfortunately,
it's *me* who practices yoga and *he* who practices standing!
Unable to come to a full stand, his legs gave way and he
dropped to the perfect "baby crawl" position, once again
mobile and a little less frustrated.

"Buddy!" I called out.

On hands and knees, his head turned around toward
me. He recognized my voice unquestionably. His almond-
shaped eyes, brown and loving, were as wide as could be,
and a grin shone brightly on his face. *What, Mommy?* his
eyes asked.

I experienced a connection so rich that my laughter was
all that held back the tears. His smile was a magnet to me
and I reached out for him. At the same time he maneuvered

himself to a seated position facing me — his arms extended, reaching out for me. We giggled together as I whisked him up and we twirled around and around.

He had been well for nearly six months. Of course, he was still on constant oxygen, had the G-tube (its use was purely for administering medicines), was diagnosed with chronic sinusitis, was in danger of pulmonary hypertension and was buying time for the inevitable heart surgery. Oh yeah, and there was that diagnosis of Down syndrome, too! All that aside, he was thriving, crawling, eating, communicating, developing and, most importantly, playing!

"It's your birthday today, Buddy," I said gasping. We plopped down to the floor, "fifteen months on the nose!" He peered curiously into my mouth as I spoke. *Maybe he'll be a dentist when he grows up!* "Happy Birthday!" I exclaimed. We were rolling on the floor and I listened to him laughing helplessly under my tickling fingers!

"Phew, I'm beat, Buddy," I said, calming down, "What about you?" We nestled together on the futon, snuggling up with a good book: *The Foot Book* by his favorite author, Dr. Seuss.

Dinner would wait.

CHAPTER NINETEEN

A 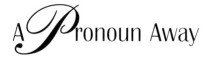ronoun Away

December 19, 1994

"Line sixty for Kim Thompson, Kim, line sixty," blared over the paging system throughout the office.

I picked up the receiver. "Hi, this is Kim. Can I help you?" I asked politely.

"Hey, it's me," my husband replied cheerfully.

It was our midday check-in call to share the morning's events. He was excited about an upcoming photo shoot for the American Cancer Society and wanted to tell me the latest news. It was to be in black and white—great for his artistic flair. When he finished telling me about the photo shoot, it was my turn to chat about the morning's work activities. Finally it was time for both of us to get back to work.

"I better go. See you tonight! Bye," I said, rushed to hang up.

"Oh, Margarite was here today. She can't believe how GREAT he's doing. She was thrilled about his standing from a kneeling position and holding himself up along the sofa."

Margarite was Buddy's cognitive therapist. Her job was to track his development and give us new goals to achieve and exercises to practice. Mostly what she loved doing was playing with Eric and creating toys for him, like the touch book she brought a couple of months ago. She pasted together different materials and created a sailboat cruising along on plastic bubble wrap ocean, a butterfly flapping its brilliant felt wings, and a fuzzy yarn teddy bear with a red ribbon bow. Inside all of this artistry, Buddy was learning.

"Oh, yeah, I forgot she was coming. What did she work on with him today?" I asked.

"She worked on his drinking with a sippy cup and practiced standing from a seated position."

"Did he drink out of the sippy cup?"

"Yeah, about three ounces," he answered like a proud dad.

"Great!" I said. "I've got to go."

"Oh, wait," he said solemnly.

"What!" I begged, now alarmed.

He paused for a moment. I heard something in that silence that dredged up that familiar fear that lurked behind every door and around every corner. "What is it?" I asked, again slightly desperate.

"Their baby died," he announced.

My heart fell as my body slouched; the muscle tone that normally kept my body erect let go. *Did he say "our"? No, no, he said "their;" but "their" is so close to our, he could just as easily have said our.* The fear turned to sadness and it surged through me, starting in my throat and gushing to my ankles. Fear and sadness are a peculiar pair. First the fear creates an adrenaline rush, tightening, contracting, flooding out of control, then sadness follows, consuming, draining and gradually eroding the spirit bit by bit.

"Whose baby?" I asked impatiently.

"Annie and Mike's," he answered, awaiting my reaction.

I was silent a moment, letting the emotions take over. The knot in my throat kept me from speaking. He knew. He'd heard this silence before. My mind raced back, into my past, where death did not occur to those who were close to me, and I was left with nothing to do, nowhere to go and nothing to say. I experienced an emotion that I never knew existed. I was stricken with empathy: pure, raw empathy. I had just seen their daughter, Samantha, less than two months ago at the *Up with Downs* meeting. She was six months old and fully recovered from the emergency heart surgery she had endured two months prior. By our request, her mom, Annie, openly showed us Samantha's two-inch-long, pink scar running down the middle of her chest to just above her bellybutton. It was an inspiration to watch Mike hold his healthy-looking, pink baby, crying, eating and sleeping while he talked about the surgery as being "quite an experience." They were over it, and my relief and happiness for them was ashamedly clouded by envy. We *weren't* over it.

I thought back to the day she had called me.

"Hi, my name is Annie Swanson. I was given your name by Karen Dearoff."

I knew immediately why she had called. I, too, spoke with Karen the day after delivering a Down's baby. Karen began *Up with Downs* in the Tampa Bay area thirteen years ago, one year after her second child, a Down's baby, was born. She was at a point where she knew she needed more support and counted on others needing it too. She has created a reputation for herself, and every new mother of a Down's baby was given her name and number. If you didn't call her, she would call you.

At last, I was standing on the other side. Someone was calling me for support. I was no longer the person who did the calling, but, rather, the one who was called, the shoulder, the one who'd been through it. Annie was sweet on the phone and seemed to be coping much better than I had. We met for lunch and immediately connected. I gave her Margarite's number, as well as our chiropractor's, who, free of charge, had been adjusting Eric since birth. Also, I passed on a list of government agencies that support families with babies like ours.

"I'll talk to you later," I said somberly to Bob. I allowed the wave of emotions to pass and all I could envision was her face at lunch with that bouncy, blond hair and the black and white polka-dotted bow pinned at the top, so innocent looking, yet not. I haven't purposefully said a prayer since Easter at Catholic Mass when I was seven, maybe eight, years old, but I sat quietly at my desk for a few minutes and whispered a prayer for her. I thought she could use one about now. As my head bowed, I felt the cool drop of a tear splash onto my hand.

CHAPTER TWENTY

Home Away from *H*ome, Part II

January – December 1994

- Jan 1   Eric was still in the hospital with pneumonia
- Jan 2   Eric was discharged
- Jan 12   Eric was admitted with a 104-degree temperature, low oxygen saturation and pneumonia in the right lung
- Jan 18   A cardiac catheterization was performed, which is an exploratory surgery to determine the urgency of heart surgery
- Jan 19   A bronchoscopy was performed (a surgical procedure to view Eric's constricted airway)
- Jan 21   Eric was discharged
- Jan 31   Eric was admitted for respiratory syncitial virus (RSV, an often fatal lung virus) and rotovirus (an intestinal virus)
- Feb 5   Eric was discharged
- Apr 20   Eric had minor surgery to insert tubes into his ears (hearing improved considerably after this surgery)
- May 12   Eric was admitted with a high fever,

low oxygen saturation, pneumonia, resistance to eating and sinusitis

- May 17   Eric was discharged
- Oct 28   Eric was admitted for a hearing test and a CAT scan of his sinuses
- Dec 6   Eric was admitted with his second bout of RSV
- Dec 11   Eric was discharged
- Dec 28   Eric had a follow-up hearing test (determined that Eric had a slight impairment in the left ear only in a certain frequency range)
- Dec 28   Eric was discharged

As Long As We Have Him

January 1995, two weeks before heart surgery...

"Is he French or Spanish?" I asked Bob as Dr. Leroud (pronounced le-rue) stepped out of the examination room.

"Spanish," he said confidently. " Listen to his accent, it comes out on certain words."

The doctor re-entered the room, sat down across from us and immediately launched into a monologue.

"You know, I can't believe it's been twenty years since I graduated from med school. I came into this practice when society was still allowing Down's babies to be institutionalized, and we had no technology to correct heart problems like his."

He turned his focus toward Eric, who was tearing apart the paper sheet draped over the examination table. Peering over the top of his eyeglasses, he continued.

"Last year we performed many heart surgeries, roughly 250, and in doing so many, we're getting better and better. We have a team made up of two intensivists, three cardiologists and two surgeons. We hold a conference every Monday to discuss cases and determine our recommendation for each patient's treatment. No one person can decide, we work together. We'll look at the results of the catheterization data and his echocardiograms from last January to see what the next step is."

As the doctor continued, I listened, comforted by Eric's sleepful hum as he rested peacefully now against my chest. I tightened my embrace as the doctor kept talking.

"If he doesn't have surgery he'll eventually die of heart disease. It's gradual and slow and the whole family suffers. Fixed pulmonary hypertension will develop and worsen, thereby restricting the blood flow to his lungs. A bluish sheen will begin to tint his skin, and as the years go by, the color will deepen. He'll gradually lose energy as his lungs will weaken. Afternoon naps will grow longer and playtime will shorten. Out of sheer exhaustion, he won't last through a session of physical therapy. Finally, in ten or fifteen years, when his immune system has weakened considerably, he'll catch a virus or develop pneumonia and not be able to fight it off. Maybe his lungs will just give out."

This was the harsh reality, the ugly truth, delivered to us by a guy we met just 20 minutes earlier. I had never heard this possible future before, never mind spoken quite so morbidly and eloquently. His bedside manner continued to plummet, but he was, at least, the most straightforward doctor we'd yet encountered.

He clarified his opinion in case we didn't get the point. "If it were my child, I'd rather have him die a thousand times on the operating table rather than the slow, agonizing death of heart disease."

I sat staring, almost in a trance, as I lightly ran my shaking fingers through Eric's hair.

"There's a risk," he went on (*does he ever stop?*), "as in all open-heart surgeries. Whether ten percent or twenty-five percent, though, what are the choices? We can at least give him a chance and, God willing, give him a full life." He paused a moment waiting for his words to come crashing down on us. "Yes, it's risky, but the alternative is, well, as I said, it would be a rough life for all of you."

He was clear and confident even in the uncertainty of it all. I despised his candor, and yet I was thankful for it. He was uncaring and detached and at the same time committed to saving my baby's life. He was like a mechanic, only Eric's body was made of flesh and the engine beat rhythmically. I sat in awe listening to him, wondering what kind of super-human material his own heart was made of that gave him the strength to endure watching sick babies come and sick babies go.

Bob spoke after an awkward silence. "Thank you for your honesty and clarity. We haven't gotten much of that over the past year."

"Communication," Dr. Leroud stated, "is what will get you through this bad time."

He's dubbed this time in our life "bad" thank you. Just maybe, maybe, it's the best year of my life. I've been more alive and more in love with life than ever before. It's the first year of my life with a new being, someone I was a partner in creating. A human being. Someone who can inspire me with a simple smile or a hearty laugh. Bad time? No, good doctor, it's just a pity not everyone could experience the remarkable time that I've had.

"Just be sure to come to one of the cardiologists or sur-geons with your questions. Don't ask whoever happens to be at Eric's bedside—try not to get caught in the minutiae."

"We've been wrapped up in that before," Bob said adding, "asking questions of whoever was close by: a nurse, a respiratory therapist, another parent, anyone."

"That would be very upsetting," he replied.

I nodded in agreement. "It was."

"It's like watching the dividing lines on the road while

you're driving," the doctor said. "You can't see where you're going and you'll soon veer off and hit a tree or a person. Keep your eyes out in front of the car and keep looking at the big picture." He nodded, pleased with his analogy.

Although his words woke me up to the severity of the surgery, he spoke of death too often for my sensitive ears. I winced at the recollection of the sharpness of his tone when he first blatantly said "die," while my heart beckoned for some reassurance.

"He's not unusual," he said, as if hearing my thoughts.

Maybe this is all routine, and because it happened to us it only seems unique?

I kissed the top of my napping baby's head and gingerly patted his back as he slept quietly.

No, this moment is special.

As we walked to the Jeep, the forty-seven-degree chill rushed up my jacket and down my back. I kissed Buddy's cheek as Bob lifted him from me.

"One thing I realized from that visit..."

"Mmm, hmm," he uttered, strapping Buddy into his car seat.

"We'll have him as long as we have him, and that's as long as we'll have him."

CHAPTER TWENTY-TWO

In the 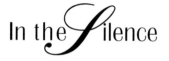ilence

January 15, 1995, Sunday

We called, sent faxes, mailed invitations, grocery shopped, rearranged furniture, borrowed chairs, cooked and baked all night and, at 11 a.m., Sunday, January 15, 1995, the day before Eric was to be admitted to the hospital, they came. Thirty, forty or fifty people piled into our house, bringing with them bagels and lox, fruit salad, quiche, croissants, Buffalo wings, champagne and their love.

They came from Michigan, California, Connecticut, Georgia and cities and towns throughout Florida. Aunt Arline, with her touch of elegance, wafted in with a concerned laugh, a warm hug and a jug of Chardonnay. Behind her followed her dad, my Pepe. As resilient as they come, he had his oxygen tank slung over his shoulder and his hearing aid turned up! I greeted him with a framed picture of Eric and him that Bob had taken at Christmas, both of them with their oxygen canulas strung across their faces. My handsome Latin friend, Ernie, who had been with us the day I delivered Eric, and whom I'd known since the Air Force days, strolled in with his boyfriend after a relaxing morning at the beach. Genie and Mark shuffled in cautiously, careful not to spill the Crockpot full of Genie's special Thai soup. Artists, psychologists, accountants and writers came; some quiet, some loud. They chatted about topics ranging from the unusual coolness of the day to their careers, the holidays and always, Eric.

A few hours passed, the "brunch pourri" was a hit, the glasses filled earlier with mimosas were empty, the third pot of coffee was cold and a few people had departed. The day was winding down.

I heard Bob in the Florida room booming, "Could everyone come into the living room, please?" He opened the sliding glass doors and yelled the same to those outside. I knew what he was doing; we had argued about it earlier. I didn't want everyone to gather together to openly acknowledge the reason they had all come; I wanted to keep the day light, full of fun, food and drink; a celebration of life. I wasn't ready to open my heart, to face the coming week... I just wasn't ready.

Everyone except me—with my secret adversity—squeezed into the living room.

As he looked around the room at each of our guests, Bob began. "Thank you all for coming today to be with us and to be with Eric." All eyes diverted momentarily from Bob to Eric, who was sitting on Grandma Sharon's lap playing a quiet game of pattycake. "As you know, Eric is going into the hospital tomorrow. He'll have a cardiac catheterization Tuesday morning, which will confirm that his heart and lungs are in a healthy enough state to withstand heart surgery. The actual surgery is scheduled for Thursday morning."

I sneaked sheepishly into the living room from the kitchen. After a moment, seeing the acceptance in the room, I decided to stay.

"I'd like to ask everyone to focus your energy on Eric and visualize his successful surgery, speedy recovery and complete health. If you don't mind, could we spend a minute being silent: thinking, praying, meditating, sending your energy to Eric, whatever it is you do. Could we be silent for a moment for Eric?" Bob bowed his head. Most closed their eyes and some bowed with him.

I looked around the room honoring the people who were partaking so willingly in this gathering for Buddy. I stopped short noticing two sets of parental eyes, wide open, staring directly at me... deep into me. They were penetrating eyes, behind which I sensed some anxiety and empathy, but mostly love. It was the kind of love that filled my body, that was responsible for my being here, that stayed with me no matter where I went or what I did. It was an infinite love I sensed, one that only parents could give. The tears welled up in my eyes, acknowledging their love. I looked over at Eric and envisioned a translucent light beam connecting us, three generations of us, allowing healing energy—love—to pass between us.

"Thank you." Bob spoke peacefully, breaking the silence. "I'd like to read a poem Stacy wrote for Eric and for everyone here." He put his hand on her shoulder... "it's called *In the Silence.*

>*At certain times, we have thoughts*
>*We're afraid to even think.*
>*Afraid that their escape into words*
>*May make them true.*
>*The "what ifs" that cannot be allowed,*
>*Though we have them, all of us,*
>*Secretly struggling to be kept silent."*

Listening to the words, I let my mind float back in time...

Eric was perhaps three weeks old. We had had nurses' visits daily to check his vital signs, listen to his heart and lungs, take blood samples and support and train us in taking care of our baby. Our two-bedroom apartment had turned into an in-home ICU.

A pregnant nurse showed up one day. *I'll bet she'll have a healthy baby* resentfully slipped into my thoughts before I could stop it.

"Hi, I'm Debbie. Where's the baby?" she asked. I showed her to the living room, where Eric was sleeping peacefully in his cradle. She lifted him gently and walked with him to the changing table in his bedroom. I followed. She immediately began pinching his skin, legs, arms and tummy.

"This baby is dehydrated. When was the last time he ate?" His little heart didn't have the energy to keep him breathing and sucking. He kept falling asleep after a few minutes of eating.

Without hesitation, she said, "Take him to the emergency room, I'll call the doctor."

"And soon, too soon,
Though we've waited for so long,
We have to give our little heart —
The one we love so much —
Into the care of medicine —
Something of which we know little
And can control even less.

"We have to watch only, and wait and hope
And struggle with our thoughts' insistent whispers.

Stand silently by and plead for someone
Bigger than ourselves to do our wish."

I remembered back to when I held him completely still so as not to disrupt any of the tubes or trigger the monitors. I wondered if this is what motherhood felt like, sitting in a hospital room, holding my baby for five minutes, maybe, if the nurse was not too fearful, pleading in my heart to let him live. I would sing quietly to him over and over again: *"You are my sunshine, my only sunshine. You make me happy, when skies are grey. You'll never know, dear, how much I love you. Please don't take my sunshine away."*

"And yet, as we stand silent,
We stand not alone.
We stand side by side with one another,
Joined in love,
With our little heart.

In the silence,
We are not idle watchers,
Or solely wishers.
We are love.
Love giving power and strength,
And peace."

I looked around the room as Bob read on. The people in the room were moved by the love we were sharing. Tears

rolled down many faces. I no longer resisted my own opening up to the love and generosity that filled my living room,
my heart.

"We trust the doctor.
The doctor trusts us.
Most of all,
We trust our little heart.
And we need no hope —
We know this heart.
It's too much a part of ours.
We've seen its power.
It's in our lives.
When we've been torn apart,
It's brought us together.

And seeing this,
We can say now, we are afraid.
We don't want to say goodbye.
We can't.
It's okay to say these words now,
They won't hurt our heart,
They are just our thoughts.

And with our thoughts now free, we wonder
Why a heart so special,
Would have to go through so much;
Why a heart so perfect,
Would need to be repaired.

And we think of how this one little heart

Has repaired so many of ours,
In so many ways, between so many people.
Perhaps, we must return the favor now
The only way we can.
Yes, of course, we're still scared
And want to hold onto our little heart,
Just the way he is.
We can't help but think,
Maybe now is not the time."

Just two months ago we had made the decision. "Yes, let's do it now while he's healthy," I had said to Bob while waiting for the doctor to return. *While he was healthy,* I thought, *I'm going to put my baby's life in jeopardy. How could I do that?* It was a decision no parent should ever have to make. Eric had been off the oxygen only two weeks, finally strong enough to sustain his own breath. He crawled, and sat up straight, and laughed and played. No pneumonia or sinusitis had weakened him for over a month. It was time. The doctors recommended we not wait because of the growing risk of pulmonary hypertension (hardened lungs, as I understood it), which could complicate or even prevent heart surgery—a condition that, in and of itself, would eventually kill him.

"Okay, let's do it now," Bob agreed.

We then scheduled Eric's hospital admission, an echocardiogram, a cardiac catheterization, the heart surgery and a brunch. The brunch was Bob's idea. His parents would be in town visiting from California anyway, and we both knew we needed to be surrounded by people who loved us, now more than ever.

And yet somehow, we think,
He didn't listen to us
When we told him
Our hearts were not ready to mend.

And now we know our part —
Once again this little heart reminds us —
Our part is love.

And as we stand by those days,
As we all will,
Wherever we happen to be,
In the silence,
Our hearts will hear his whisper
And we will know.
He is not done reminding us
Of many, many things.

And so together and alone,
We will wait and hope and love.
But quietly, thankfully, we'll know.
Our little heart will beat.

The Day 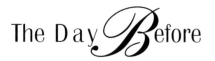efore

January 18, 1995

I awoke deeply consumed by negative thoughts. I resisted, but they came against my will, taunting me, intensifying the fear that had already paralyzed me. *What will I do if he doesn't make it? Will the sounds of a laughing baby bring sadness? Would we have another baby, could another baby ever measure up to what we have in Eric?* The noise flooded my mind as even more nightmarish scenarios played themselves out; the handsome Doctor V. (his Indian heritage gave him a last name that is tough for most Westerners to pronounce), Eric's surgeon, walks toward us, not in his usual beaming doctor manner, but slower, head cocked to one side, eyelids lowered. He says, "I'm so sorry." The image brings with it a sense of melting from inside out, no tears or hysterics, just melting.

I had no energy to fight off these horrible fantasies, so I laid there like a victim, quiet and still, letting my mind take over. The knock on the door pulled me out of the blackness where I was dwelling. "It's seven o'clock, time to get up," Jonathan called through the door.

The thoughts scattered and hid as I yelled back, "Thanks, I'm awake!" I rolled over and hugged my sleeping husband, hoping the thoughts wouldn't find me again.

꿏

It was the first night we spent at the Clarks' home. They lived only ten minutes from the hospital where Buddy was and we didn't want to be alone in our house without him this week. Eric was admitted Monday, January 16th, with an undetermined discharge date.

"We'll see how he does," said Dr. Beals, his new cardiologist, when we asked how long Eric would be in the hospital. He was scheduled for a cardiac catheterization at 7 a.m. Tuesday morning. We went in early to be with him. I held him as his body went limp from the pre-anesthesia sedative. I anguished silently as they lifted him, groggy and helpless, from my shoulder. They requested we remain in the waiting room. The strength I kept rebuilding waned once again.

After two and a half hours of drinking coffee, dozing, staring at magazine advertisements and trying not to pay attention to my racing mind, Dr. Beals suddenly plopped into the chair next to me. I nudged Bob awake. I'd only met this man twice before, but as far as I could sense, he wasn't emitting a very positive air. Expressionless, he began reporting his findings.

"As you know, we did the cath so we would have a clear picture of Eric's heart defect and how his lungs have been affected by it. It turns out it's as I had suspected. The arterial pressures in his lungs are very high, about double the norm. Probably not so high that Dr. V. won't do the surgery, but high enough that we can't be sure the pulmonary hypertension is reversible, which means the lungs may not adapt to the corrected heart after the surgery. He may still need to be on oxygen afterward."

"How long," I asked?

"There's no telling. I'll have to show the results to Doctor

V. to make sure he'll still do the surgery."

I prayed for the surgery to happen. I recalled Doctor Beals' partner informing us of Eric's declining health and certain early death if the surgery weren't possible.

"I'm ninety-five percent sure he'll do it, but only he can say. I'll stop by Eric's bed around four this afternoon and let you know. Do you have any questions?"

We prompted him for some assurance, but were left with complete uncertainty. This unknowing and uncertainty was becoming a way of life, and I found myself searching for anything tangible to grasp.

Dr. V. himself came by that afternoon. He was concerned by the results of the cath, but his demeanor was not as heavy as his colleague's.

"The surgery is a go for Thursday morning at seven, giving him one day to recuperate from today's surgery. They'll take him down to the OR for prep at six, so if you want to see him beforehand, come earlier," he recommended.

"Are you concerned about him getting through the surgery?" I asked.

"Ninety-nine percent of the kids make it through the surgery okay. It's the following twenty-four to forty-eight hours that are critical. If he's improving by Saturday night, then he'll be fine."

It was Wednesday at 7 a.m., exactly twenty-four hours before the moment that I've been anticipating anxiously and dreading wholeheartedly for one year and five months, since Eric was two days old. I showered and dressed in sort of a shock state, left powerless after another morning of battling with my thoughts. *Would I remain in this unconscious, fore-*

boding state for the next seventy-two hours? Maybe it would be better to not be fully present during this period. Then if the worst happens, my memory would be clouded by a fog.

I was sitting on the floor of the bedroom tying my shoes, when it hit me: *I may not be a mother on Sunday.*

That one did me in, the battle had been won and I lost. Unconsciousness turned into convulsive hysteria. I wailed for every mother who has ever lost her baby, for myself, for Eric and for the treatment that he's been through and all that he would have to endure in his life. I cried for the little boy in the hospital playroom who had leukemia and for his daddy who played Pac Man with him. I was caught in an emotional tidal wave, swirling and whirling and drowning.

Some amount of time had passed when Bob walked in and found me curled on the floor with my arms wrapped around my legs. He picked me up to a seated position and wrapped his arms tightly around me. "What's going on?" he whispered tenderly.

I remained quiet for a moment, trying to regain my composure, enough, at least, to respond. "Bad thoughts... just horrible," I choked. We didn't move until I finally lifted my head and said I was okay. He understood. Bad thoughts filtered through him, also.

We finished our morning routine in silence and went out to the kitchen, where Jonathan was pouring freshly squeezed orange juice for all of us.

"Good morning!" he said cheerfully.

"Mornin'," we replied in unison.

"Anything going on?" he asked. A heaviness fell, almost audible.

I was speechless. Bob answered hesitantly, "We're scared."

Jonathan closed the refrigerator door and turned toward

us, asking, "Are you talking? Are you saying to each other everything that you're thinking?"

"I think so," I answered sheepishly.

"I don't think so," he said back. "Let's sit down and talk."

I didn't want to. I wanted to go see my baby and I wasn't up to confronting this morning's attackers. I knew a conversation with him would have me do just that.

He coaxed us into the living room and I sat at the furthest point from Jonathan and Bob, which was also the closest seat to the door, just in case I wanted to escape. I decided I would let Bob talk. I would just listen, keeping myself out the conversation. They both looked at me from across the room and Jonathan patted the cushion between them as if to say, "Come sit here, won't you?"

Damn, he caught me. I arose slowly, shuffled over to them and sat quietly down.

"Bob actually looks okay, and you don't. What are you thinking?" Jonathan asked me.

I looked beyond him out through their patio and out onto the golf course. I wished I were the bird out there chirping away, not a care in the world, or one of the palm trees, or that I could meld into the rolling green hills. Hell, I wished I were the golf cart, anything but who I was or where I was.

"Come back here," he said. "What are you thinking?"

I spoke after a few minutes. "Besides wishing that I weren't here..." I lightened up for a brief moment—not really.

"What else?" he persisted.

My eyes welled. The thoughts came out of hiding, but the words were caught in my throat.

"I don't want to say" was what came out.

His eyes pierced into mine.

I took a deep breath, and another. My mouth opened, but this time nothing came out.

"What's there to say?" he asked.

Shut up. Leave me alone. Go away. I hate you. "I'm afraid," I uttered under my breath.

"Of what?"

Pause. "Afraid I won't be a mother on Sunday." The tears streamed down my cheeks, as I held my head in my hands.

"You'll always be a mother," he responded, "no matter what happens tomorrow, or Friday, or Saturday, or in the next thirty years. You can't not be a mother. You already are one."

"But, what if... ," my voice trailed off under my breath as my gaze drifted back to his eyes.

"There is no what if, you are a mother now and forever, whether Eric makes it through the surgery or not."

He said more, but the words were no longer clear. I was sweating profusely, which seemed like a release of pent up anxiousness. The negative thoughts dissipated as he continued to speak, looking directly into my eyes. I was lightening up, letting go of what I conceded would be with me for some time. I became clearer in the conversation, which continued for another half hour, until finally there was truly nothing more to say. I was ready to be with Eric, to be with him in a way that would have our lives be fulfilled and in love today, regardless of what tomorrow would bring.

Will of the 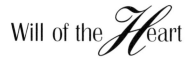eart

January 19, 1995, Thursday, 17 months after birth

"Good morning, Buddy," I whispered as I reached for his limp hand through the steel bars. It was 5 a.m, two hours before surgery and one hour before they would cart him away to administer the initial anesthesia and take care of whatever prep work needed to be done prior to open-heart surgery. As I softly stroked his tiny fingers, trying not to wake him and, at the same time, hoping that he would awaken, I pondered in awe that my life had brought me to this point. The days of "it only happens to other people" have been long gone, but somehow the implausibleness of it all crept back into my consciousness as I stared at the figure lying helpless, seemingly unaware of what was about to transpire. I studied his figure intently, emblazoning the vision of his form into my memory. I was afraid I might forget.

"I want to hold him," I whispered to Bob across the darkened room.

"I don't think we can," he whispered back, looking up at me. I saw the shimmer of a tear in his eye reflecting off the light in the hallway.

I was sad for him, remembering the first conversation we ever had about children. I was twenty-two and he was twenty-three, only a year into our relationship. At that point, I never thought I would have children; mothering didn't call to me. Having children was a concept I said I would maybe think about in ten years. But Bob knew he wanted to father a baby during his lifetime. He said he would like to have a boy, so that he could cheer for him at Little League games, be the proud father in the stands and take him to pro baseball games, things like that. But he wasn't bound to having a boy—it was a baby he knew he wanted. I was taken aback by his confidence in knowing exactly how he felt about having a child and warmed by his sharing this feeling with me. That was nearly ten years ago.

I carefully released the knobs on the crib and the side dropped down with a clang. Luckily, the baby only stirred, but the nurse came flying into the room.

"I was going to try to hold him," I offered before she could scold me.

"Let me help you," she said, rounding the crib. She untied the cloth from around his wrist, which bound him to the crib, keeping him from loosening the IV. Then she detached the oxygen saturation monitor and the pulse oximeter. She slipped one hand under his neck, cupped his behind with the other hand, and lifted. Standing on the opposite side of the crib, I accepted his body into my arms, trying to steady myself. I couldn't pull him close to me, the oxygen tube was not long enough. I was holding him, leaning over the crib trying to get close enough to feel the warmth of his body and the softness of his skin against my own. My arms began shaking from the weight. Light as he was, the awkward stance offered no leverage, so I finally had to put him down. I touched my cheek to his and whispered. "I love you. I'm here for you," into his ear and laid him back down. *So frustrating not to be able to do such a normal thing*

*as hold my baby... too intense... I'm not ready for this...
please don't let this really be happening.*

We took over the couch in the waiting room that faced
the entrance from the hallway, so we could watch for the
doctor. It was so cold in there; the room was further chilled
by the faces that occupied the other chairs and couches. I
closed my eyes, desperately begging for sleep to come; I
wanted to escape, fall into another time, another land. But
the comfort of sleep never came. It was far too cold and the
fearful thoughts were far too dominant.

"Would you like some coffee?" the volunteer asked yank-
ing me out of my own mind.

"Thank you, yes," I answered, surrendering to wakeful-
ness.

It was 6:50 a.m. when a nurse, outfitted in hospital
greens, topped with what looked like a shower cap,
approached us. "The doctor will begin at 7 a.m. Eric is all
prepped and doing fine. The surgery should take about four
hours, and I'll come back out around nine to let you know
how everything is going."

I nodded, looking up at her. There was nothing to say at
this point.

*What is this fog I'm in? This isn't real. Who is this
woman? Why am I here? What is this horrible feeling inside
that I can't get rid of? Why am I shaking? I want to scream,
stop time, make everyone stop talking to me like everything is
just fine, rip out this dreadful feeling...!* My mind was racing
wildly. I couldn't control it. *Okay, deep breaths.* Tears. *Deep
breaths.* More tears. *Deep breaths.* The tears subsided. *Deep
breaths.* I could open my eyes. *Deep breaths.* I could speak

again.

"Let's go outside," I suggested to Bob. I had no energy to listen to what was going on inside of him. I could tell by the look on his face he was also becoming lost in fearful thoughts. We held hands walking together and we stayed close to each other all day. What we were experiencing was personal, individual. Eric was my only child and he was Bob's only child. The relationship we had with Eric was our own: The pain, the despair, the joy and love, although shared between our three souls, lived distinctly inside each of us.

An hour later...

"Hi, Stace!" Bob exclaimed as she walked into the waiting room. I lifted my head from his shoulder and opened my eyes.

How beautiful she is, I thought at first glance. I was glad to see her and thankful for her warm smile and loving, empathetic eyes. Her angelic, golden glow seemed out of place in this room. Beaming was not how I would have described the other faces in there.

"Thanks for coming," I said as she reached out to hug me. She wiped her own tears away as she sat down beside me. She was Buddy's best friend, not to mention his biggest fan. They had a special relationship that I'll never know, but that was fine with me. I was able to witness the love they shared, and I figured, the more love out there the better off everyone will be.

"Are you guys doing okay?" she asked.

There was no way to really answer that question. It did, however, start us talking, which it seemed time to do. We shared with her and each other all the thoughts and feelings that had come up, as well as rehashing the events of the morning. Dressed for work and on her way there, she was only going to stay an hour. "Work" never saw her that day; she stayed with us.

"The doctor has opened him up and is now patching his heart. He's doing well," the same green-clad nurse informed us at the 9 a.m check-in. "The doctor will be out when it's over." And she was gone as quickly as she had arrived.

More coffee, more talking, more tension as we waited....

I spotted Doctor V. standing at the doorway and looked down at my watch. It was 12:13 p.m. *Here it is*, I thought, *the moment of truth, when my life will go either this way or that, a crossroads leading to two different futures, both unpredictable, both unknown...*

Standing before us in his clean white robe, a straight-faced Doctor V. said, "The surgery was successful and Eric is doing well. He's in recovery right now for the next two hours. You can see him at the 3 p.m. visit. I'll meet you by his bedside at 4 p.m. We can talk more then."

The tenseness throughout my body relaxed. It was like a drug had just been injected into me and soothing relief was flooding my veins. I've never experienced such a sensation before; my future had seemed to weigh so completely on his words.

125

"Thank you," I said to the doctor with every bit of sincerity that has ever existed in the world. Those two words seemed too trivial to say to a man who had just saved my baby's life. I wanted to tell him how much I appreciated that he spent so many years in school studying and learning how to perform surgery, that the world was a better place because of him, that his dedication and commitment to saving lives was beyond extraordinary.

I wanted to spring from my chair and sprint down the hall, slam open the doors and take in the sights and sounds of the world from "the other side," a place where I was now standing — post-surgery. "Let's get out of here," I exclaimed slightly out of breath, "Let's go for a walk."

"Go!" Stacy cried out to Bob and me. "I want to call Jonathan."

Hand in hand, we raced down the corridor and out the front door. We walked fast, very fast, up this street, down that path, through the park, noticing all the wild daisies and pansies and Spanish moss dripping over the pavement, amused by the geckos that scattered out of our way. We talked about the colors of nature, and acknowledged the incredibly gorgeous day. But mostly, we wallowed in the intense love we were both feeling and the exhilaration of a new future that had just begun.

The doctor was waiting for us beside Eric's bed. His face read success, but I was aghast at the sight of my baby. The number of tubes that flowed from Eric's body reminded me of Frankenstein's monster: two thin black wires strung out from his sternum, connecting the pacemaker to a black box that rested on his tummy; two thick yellowish, ten-foot-long tubes clogged with blood reached out of his chest and down to a tank that collected the liquid draining from his heart; the familiar blue breathing tube jammed down his throat pumped air into his lungs; the heplock block that was attached to his temple and allowed the nurses to extract blood without having to stick him every time and nourish him with the clear fluid from the IV drip; the white band that was wrapped tightly around his big toe on such a tiny foot stretched down the length of the bed to the device that measured his oxygen saturation level; and finally the alarming beeps, buzzes and hum of monitors encircled his crib.

Dressed in cheery plum scrubs and stationed at the foot of the bed, a nurse sat on a swivel chair and bent over a table, apparently notating Eric's condition.

"Hi, I'm Pat," she said with a broad, plum-lipped smile, looking up from her forms, "I'll be Eric's nurse during the 12-hour day shift."

I shot her a hesitant smile then turned my attention back to my son.

"He's stable, but we'll be keeping a close watch on him through the weekend," said Dr. V., "the next 48 hours will be crucial."

Over the next three days, Bob and I stayed next to Eric's bed in MICU (Medical Intensive Care Unit) when we were allowed and languored in the waiting room when we were asked to leave. Time passed slowly, but with every minute, Eric was regaining his energy. One by one, they pulled the tentacles out—first the wires, next, the gunky yellow tubes, then the breathing hose and finally the odd-looking clear and silver appendage connected to his head.

The pale blue hospital blanket was folded down to below his belly-button warming from his legs to his toes. His chest bore multiple scars from a battle, but five days had passed and he was the victor. The three inch vertical wound separated the right side of his torso from the left, pointing upward, where a wide smile crossed his face as he watched his mommy watching him. His sleepy eyes looked up at me as if to say, "I did it!" I embraced his soul through the gaze into his eyes. Only love was present. My life had begun again.

The Forty-seventh 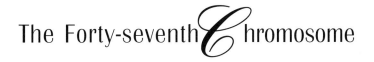 Chromosome

February 1995, one month after surgery

I wrote an ending to this story that spoke of love and miracles, creating adventures and having fun in life. This is what I learned over the past year and a half of Eric's precious life, and this is why I thought I wrote this book. I showed the ending to, Stacy, my writing partner who sat beside me on the beach Sunday after Sunday as I wrote and who had listened to my story word for word.

With a Cheshire cat grin, wallowing in self-satisfaction, I read the closing aloud to her. I thought I had found the answer. I thought I had reached the other side, that my transformation was truly over.

After hearing the words of my enlightenment and how I had become more aware and alive, her response was "What's underneath all of that?"

"Underneath what?" I asked defensively, resisting her intuition. I couldn't answer. I thought I had reached the TRUTH. I know she listened from her heart, but didn't I write from the same place? I found the "answer," no matter what she said. She was wrong this time. But what did she mean? Why did she ask me that question when she knew my soul was in those words? I was sure I was complete, that this year was a time of growth for me with Eric as my

teacher and our circumstances as his tools. Her question
weighed heavily on my mind. I couldn't help but inquire as
to what might lie beneath my incomplete truth.

The following Sunday, I was strolling aimlessly down the
aisles of Barnes & Noble, catching glimpses of this Zen book
and that cookbook, not focusing on any particular one. I
was preoccupied. My mind remained fixated on my friend's
probing question from last week.

Suddenly, I noticed I couldn't read the names of the
books I was seeing—the letters were blurred. There was
something in my vision—it was a tear. It came to me without
warning. I dropped my writing pad and my purse fell off my
right shoulder. I stopped dead in the aisle and leaned
against the bookcase in the Philosophy section. My mind
was taken over with the vision of my Buddy. His sweet smile
opened my heart. *What was I feeling? What was happening
to me?* I was calm, yet elated. I felt relaxed and at the same
time so wound up I wanted to run wildly. I sensed freedom
flowing through my veins, *but freedom from what*, I wondered. It wasn't the freedom of an escape, it was more like a
release from bondage. *What bondage, though?* I didn't move,
I didn't see any people or books or bookcases, all I could
envision were Eric's sparkling eyes as I watched him giggle
at me.

I heard it clearly through his silent laughter. I was my
own bondage. I held my heart captive and wouldn't allow it
to love him unconditionally, as mothers do. I kept myself far
enough away, a safe distance, just in case. *In case of what?*
In case he hadn't made it through his heart surgery, in case
he started looking too Down's-like, in case I didn't want to
deal with people's whispers, in case... in case I never wanted
to confront my fear of unconditionally loving my baby.

I was afraid, afraid to love someone unconditionally. It

had seemed vulnerable and weak, inconceivable, actually, to love that openly, that freely, but somehow it wasn't that at all. It was strengthening! I was exhilarated! This love, he taught me, did not even have to be directed to just one person, but to anyone, everyone. My heart raced as my breathing quickened. It all made sense. His Down syndrome was a gift, a gift to me and maybe, God willing, a gift to everyone. I smiled a knowing smile as cleansing tears fell from my eyes. *This is what the forty-seventh chromosome is filled with... love... unconditional love. This is Eric's gift.*

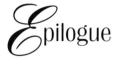

Epilogue

August 15, 1995, one week before Eric's second birthday

His giggles echo in my heart as he teases us with the teal cloth placemat, wrapping it around his head like a bonnet and then covering his face. We play along willingly, saying aloud, "Where's Buddy? Where did Buddy go?" on and on until he decides to pull the placemat down from his face and show us his bright eyes and beaming smile. He's laughing uproariously at us for falling for his peekaboo game every time. He does this six, maybe seven, times in a row and we play along every time, until, finally, he moves on to a new game.

I think it's appropriate that this book is nearly complete because I'm writing from a different "place" now. I've turned down the road and am now living in that unexpected future of which I was once so frightened. It is a future full of possibilities that I get to create every moment. Leaping into the unknown can be risky and frightening, but the joy and exhilaration while in flight makes it all worthwhile. With that 'aliveness' comes a sense of tranquillity that keeps me grounded and at peace. Writing has been a part of the past two years through my grieving, growing, healing, learning and loving process, and now this chapter of my life is drawing to a close.

Eric is nearly two, and fully recovered from the heart surgery that took place just seven months ago. He's miraculous, my son. My son. My baby, who teetered on the edge of life too many times, who taught me the way to be true to myself, to be honest with those around me and to express love unconditionally.

I watch his way of being. He's happy, playful and loving, inspiring people as they cross his path: my parents; our friends; the cashier at the grocery store; his pediatric psychologist, who began the session stiff and direct and ended on the floor laughing and playing ball with Eric; his favorite babysitter who calls *us* to babysit; and so on. My eyes sink deep into his soul and I realize how honored I am that he chose me to be his mother. Then I graciously thank his soul. I think to myself in wonder how far I've come from those early days of "how could this have happened to me." Now, it's more like "how could this not have happened to me." A very dear friend of mine once spoke a cliché to me when I was an impressionable sixteen-year-old: "God never gives you what you can't handle." Well, I'm still developing my relationship with God and exploring spirituality, as well as inquiring into that which lies deep inside each of us, connecting all of us. But, she was right and I, we handled it and will continue to handle the circumstances that arise while being thankful for every one of them.

During my pregnancy, before any of the future events portrayed in this book were ever known, Bob and I created a context for our family: our life purpose. We put into words that inner desire that I believe everyone possesses, which is to contribute to the world, to make a profound difference with people. Our family, from that day forward, in everything we said and everything we experienced, was to *inspire love and miracles.* This book, the many songs that Bob's written and shared, our family relationship, Buddy's strength and healthiness, we say are a direct result of our commitment.

In other families, people experience emotional disorders, physical handicaps, unexpected deaths, racism, famine, world wars and so much more. We have Down syndrome. How very fortunate, we are. We will all always strive to have Buddy reach his fullest potential in life, just like any other parent, I surmise. The therapies, special schools or programs, higher health expenses, extra cognitive training, nutrition and vitamins have become a natural part of our lives to the point where they are all normal. Our lives are normal again—and at the same time extraordinary. Life has become a playground to laugh, love and play together.

I have one last thing to say that I spent hours searching for. The words didn't come easily. It is gratefulness. I am thankful, but this time it is to myself. I am thankful that I gave myself the time and space to write this story, the gentleness to allow myself to go through what I needed to go through at the pace that I needed, and the courage to share it all.

Eric's 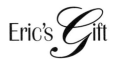ift

A poetic essay by Stacy Clark

One day a child comes into our world, bright and fresh, ready to learn and to live. We're here to take care of him and comfort him. And we stand ready to teach him all we know ourselves; to give him all we have. We're suddenly aware of all the answers to the questions we don't have yet—and he might ask. We see all the things we may be called upon to do, and wonder if we'll be ready when the time comes. And, when we look at him, just look at him, we wonder where could we have been hiding all this love all these years.

One day we notice there is more love around us since he came. And there is less anger where anger used to be. We notice we are wiser than before, and yet, strangely, we are aware we know less. People come together and bring the best of themselves to each other, and to us, since he came. Somehow life matters more—and all else matters less—since he came.

And one day we realize that he has come to us. He is teaching us and teaching us to love. And though we don't know who he'll be, our hearts forever know who he is. Always giving us all he has. Maybe, this is love. Maybe, this is Eric's Gift.

136